A Coursebook On
SCIENTIFIC AND PROFESSIONAL WRITING
for Speech-Language Pathology

Sixth Edition

A Coursebook On
SCIENTIFIC AND PROFESSIONAL WRITING
for Speech-Language Pathology

Sixth Edition

M. N. Hegde, PhD

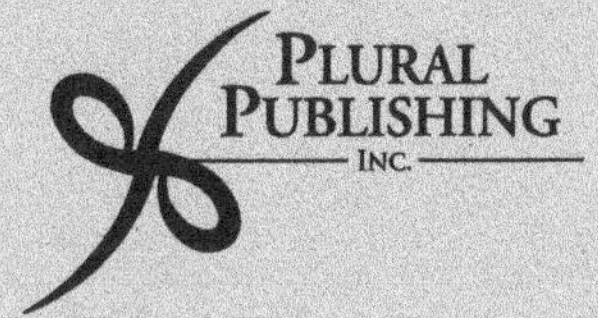

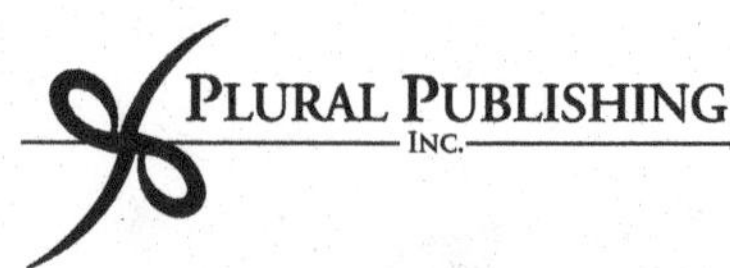

5521 Ruffin Road
San Diego, CA 92123

e-mail: information@pluralpublishing.com
Website: https://www.pluralpublishing.com

Typeset in 10.5/12 Adobe Garamond by Flanagan's Publishing Services, Inc.
Printed in the United States of America by Integrated Books International

Library of Congress Cataloging-in-Publication Data:

Names: Hegde, M. N. (Mahabalagiri N.), 1941- author.
Title: A coursebook on scientific and professional writing for speech-language pathology / M.N. Hegde, PhD, California State University - Fresno.
Description: Sixth edition. | San Diego, CA : Plural Publishing, Inc., [2024] | Includes bibliographical references and index.
Identifiers: LCCN 2022034969 (print) | LCCN 2022034970 (ebook) | ISBN 9781635504019 (spiral bound) | ISBN 9781635504026 (ebook)
Subjects: LCSH: Speech therapy—Authorship. | Medical writing.
Classification: LCC RC428.5 .H445 2024 (print) | LCC RC428.5 (ebook) | DDC 616.85/5—dc23/eng/20220802
LC record available at https://lccn.loc.gov/2022034969
LC ebook record available at https://lccn.loc.gov/2022034970

Contents

Concise and Direct Writing

Parallelism

Misplaced or Dangling Modifiers

Shifts Within and Between Sentences

Quotations

Precision in the Use of Scientific Terms

Preface to the Sixth Edition

Teaching and learning to write in a technical and professional language is an important part of education in speech-language pathology. However, students often do not begin to acquire acceptable writing skills until they enroll in clinical practicums or in graduate research seminars in which professional and scientific writing are required. Unfortunately, because of limited instruction in scientific and professional writing, many graduate students are both challenged and frustrated in their research and clinical writing assignments.

Students in speech-language pathology programs who have taken courses on writing offered in other departments still do not have adequate technical and professional writing skills. Instructors know that merely extolling good writing and asking students to read some of the many available books on how to write well are not effective. Teaching writing skills is time and effort intensive because unless students have examples to follow and receive feedback on their writing, their skills do not improve. Students have to write, receive feedback, and rewrite. Although it does not obviate the need for writing and rewriting, this coursebook makes that task somewhat more practical for both the student and the instructor.

There are many books on writing, but few give opportunities to practice writing while glancing at exemplars. Writing courses are generally designed to teach rules of grammar, not writing. An explicit knowledge of grammar rules will help avoid grammatical mistakes. But good writing goes beyond mastering grammatical rules. Also, individuals who cannot recite rules of grammar can still write well. Exemplars of good writing and opportunities to practice writing are both essential to learn writing skills. Therefore, I designed this new type of book, which I call a *coursebook.*

The most important aspect of this coursebook is the way the left-hand and right-hand pages are designed (and keyed by icons). Most left-hand pages show specific examples of general, scientific, or professional writing (eyeglass icon). In many cases, both the incorrect and correct versions are shown. The corresponding right-hand pages require the student to write correctly (pencil icon). Typically, the facing pages contain the same rules or exemplars: one to read about and the other to write on.

This coursebook is designed with the following assumptions:

- Students who simply memorize the rules of grammar do not necessarily write well; they need practice in writing.
- Students should have many examples of the skills they are expected to learn, including grammatically correct and well-organized writing using an accepted style.
- Students should read an exemplar and write one immediately.
- Students should write multiple exemplars.
- Given exemplars and the student writing should go hand in hand.
- To the extent possible, students should receive feedback in the classroom.

This book has been used in a dedicated course on scientific and professional writing. Students actually wrote in the class. Students were randomly asked to read samples of their writing. The instructor then gave feedback, correcting any mistakes. The rest of the class then corrected their mistakes, if any. This act of writing was immediately followed by positive reinforcement or corrective feedback.

It was my hope that instructors and student clinicians would find it useful in teaching and learning writing skills in the classroom. The response of instructors around the country has been overwhelmingly positive. Many instructors have commented that there has been a need for this kind of book and that the coursebook method is more effective in teaching writing skills than are traditional books on writing.

Both clinical supervisors and academic course instructors can use this book to teach scientific and professional writing skills. The book can be used in the following contexts:

- a course on writing
- courses on assessment and diagnosis
- courses on research methods and introduction to graduate studies
- clinical practicums and internships
- independent studies in writing skills
- informally assigned work to help individual students master good writing skills (students may be assigned selected sections to complete, depending on their deficiencies)

New to Sixth Edition

The scientific writing section of this sixth edition is based on the seventh edition of the *Publication Manual of the American Psychological Association* (2020). The method of citations in the text and the reference list formats have been updated to conform to the seventh edition of the *Manual.* The electronic source citation method has been updated.

Guidelines on submitting electronic papers, books, and book chapters to academic journals or publishers have been updated. How the author may manage their submitted work during the review process has also been covered. A brief overview of reviewing and revising the copyedited manuscripts, along with correcting page proofs the authors receive as PDF documents has been included. The topic of electronic submission of convention and conference proposals was updated. A revised section (B.4.62 Guidelines on Using Electronic Sources in Scientific Writing) describes safer practices of searching and evaluating web-based information for general reliability and validity. Another section (B.4.63 Examples of Electronic Sources in the Reference List) has been updated to give examples of referencing electronic sources in the reference list.

The section B.2. (Terms for Writing Without Bias) has been thoroughly revised to reflect the latest writing practices related to pronoun usage; writing without prejudicial reference to age, gender, and gender identities; varied sexual orientations, disability, ethnic or racial identity, and unfavorable comparisons of groups recruited for a research study. Several new exemplars and practice opportunities have been created for this revised edition. A new glossary that defines terms related to biased writing and appropriate alternatives has been added to this revised edition.

The professional writing section of the new edition was also revised and updated to reflect current clinical terms and practice. A new trial-by-trial treatment progress recording sheet has been added to the section on progress report writing. A Subjective, Objective, Assessment, and Plan (SOAP) progress report written in medical settings has been added to the same section. A new section has been added on report writing in public schools, which includes an assessment plan that helps determine whether a student meets the school district's criteria for enrollment in clinical speech-language services. Also included is a new SOAP document that public school clinicians may write.

Acknowledgments

I would like to thank the editorial department headed by an able editor, Valerie Johns. Her kind and continuous help is greatly appreciated. I would also like to thank Emily Pooley, the Project Editor at Plural Publishing's Editorial Department for her excellent help throughout the development process. My thanks also go to Jessica Bristow, Production Editor and Lori Asbury, Production Manager for their excellent work on this new edition. Angie Singh, the president of Plural Publishing, has been a friend and supporter for decades. I thank her and all her efficient staff at Plural Publishing.

My special thanks go to Laura Marie Brown, Speech and Language Pathologist in the Clovis Unified School District, Clovis, California. She has been an invaluable resource for me on the various kinds of reports the clinicians write in public schools. She supplied a variety of forms and guidelines that speech-language pathologists use in the educational setting. The new section on report writing in public schools reflects her expert help.

About the Author

M. N. (Giri) Hegde, PhD, Professor Emeritus of Communication Sciences and Disorders at California State University–Fresno, holds a master's degree in experimental psychology from the University of Mysore, India; a post-master's diploma in medical (clinical) psychology from Bangalore University, India; and a doctoral degree in speech-language pathology from Southern Illinois University Carbondale.

Hegde is a specialist in fluency disorders, language disorders, research methods, and treatment procedures in communicative disorders. He has made numerous presentations to national and international audiences on various basic and applied topics in communicative disorders and experimental and applied behavior analysis. With his deep and wide scholarship, Hegde has authored several highly regarded and widely used scientific and professional books, including *Clinical Research in Communicative Disorders* (with P. Salvatore), *Introduction to Communicative Disorders, A Coursebook on Aphasia and Other Neurogenic Language Disorders, Hegde's PocketGuide to Communication Disorders, Hegde's PocketGuide to Treatment in Speech-Language Pathology, Hegde's PocketGuide to Assessment in Speech-Language Pathology, Assessment of Communication Disorders in Children* (with F. Pomaville), *Assessment of Communication Disorders in Adults* (with D. Freed), *Clinical Methods and Practicum in Speech-Language Pathology* (with K. Kuyumjian), and several others. He has served on the editorial boards of scientific and professional journals and continues to serve as an editorial consultant to the *Journal of Fluency Disorders.*

Hegde is a recipient of various honors, including the Outstanding Professor Award from California State University–Fresno, California State University–Fresno Provost's Recognition for Outstanding Scholarship and Publication, Distinguished Alumnus Award from the Southern Illinois University Department of Communication Sciences and Disorders, and Outstanding Professional Achievement Award from District 5 of the California Speech-Language-Hearing Association. Hegde is a Fellow of the American Speech-Language-Hearing Association.

PART A

Foundations of Scientific and Professional Writing

A.1. Basic Rules of Usage

Ampersand

- The ampersand (&) stands for the conjunction *and.*
- It is used only with certain proper names and abbreviations.

A.1.1a. Use the Ampersand Correctly

Incorrect	Correct	Note
(Johnson and Thompson, 2022)	(Johnson & Thompson, 2022)	Two authors in parentheses or in the reference list.
American Telephone and Telegraph	American Telephone & Telegraph	Use it only if the company itself uses it.
U.S. Department of Health & Human Services	U.S. Department of Health and Human Services	Some government agencies do not use an ampersand.
The local S and L may be helpful in getting a loan.	The local S & L may be helpful in getting a loan.	Used with an abbreviation, with one space on either side of it.
The R and D spokesperson hinted at new products.	The R&D spokesperson hinted at new products.	Some technical and scientific abbreviations take an ampersand without space on either side of it.

Note: R&D refers to research and development [department].

Apostrophe

A.1.2a. Do Not Turn a Possessive Into a Plural

Use an apostrophe when needed.

Incorrect	Correct	Note
The *persons* resistance to treatment was high.	The *person's* resistance to treatment was high.	Singular possessives
The *clients* prognosis is good.	The *client's* prognosis is good.	
The *clinicians* motivation to treat matters.	The *clinicians'* motivation to treat matters.	Plural possessives
The *participants* socioeconomic status did not have an effect.	The *participants'* socioeconomic status did not have an effect.	

Ampersand

A.1.1b. Use the Ampersand Correctly

Incorrect	Write correctly
Williams and Wilkins	
Johnson and Thomson Co.	
U.S. Department of Education & Human Development	
The local S and L gives loans.	
The R and D department is nonexistent.	

Apostrophe

A.1.2b. Do Not Turn a Possessive Into a Plural

Incorrect	Write Correctly
I will train this clients mother.	
Ambiguous stimuli reduce a treatments effectiveness.	
The treatment settings influence cannot be ignored.	
Several clients progress was slow.	
The persons feelings should be considered.	
Pediatricians awareness of early language problems is limited.	

Hint: Some examples contain a plural and a possessive.

A.1.3a. Do Not Turn a Plural Into a Possessive

Do not use an unnecessary apostrophe.

Incorrect	Correct	Note
The *characteristic's* of aphasia are well known.	The *characteristics* of aphasia are well known.	Plurals, turned into possessives. Common mistakes.
The *characteristics'* of aphasia are well known.		
In the *1970's*, the clinicians began to treat language.	In the *1970s*, the clinicians began to treat language.	
I selected 10 *participants'*.	I selected 10 *participants*.	
The *animals'* have rights.	The *animals* have rights.	
Twenty *clients'* were treated.	Twenty *clients* were treated.	
The *parents'* were not cooperative.	The *parents* were not cooperative.	

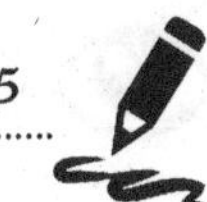

A.1.3.b. Do Not Turn a Plural Into a Possessive

Incorrect	Write Correctly
Individuals' with dysarthria have neurological problems.	
Many factors' affect the treatment outcome.	
The problems of the 1980's will persist into the 1990's.	
The clients are in their 60's.	
I studied several variables' related to the participants' language skills. *Hint:* Contains a plural and a possessive.	

A.1.4a. Use the Correct Forms of Possessive Nouns

Several rules dictate the use of possessive forms. The simplest rule is to add the apostrophe and an *s*, as in *the man's hat*, *the girl's shoes*, and *the cat's tail.* Mistakes arise from the variable practice of adding or not adding *'s* to words that end in *s*.

Incorrect	Correct	Note
The *boys's* room is large.	The *boys'* room is large.	Most regular plural words do not take an extra *s*; they only have an apostrophe.
The *ladies's* purses are small.	The *ladies'* purses are small.	
The *tigers's* look is ferocious.	The *tigers'* look is ferocious.	
The *mens* health history was not reported.	The *men's* health history was not reported.	Most irregular plurals take *'s*.
The *childrens* ages were not specified.	The *children's* ages were not specified.	
Those *womens* language skills are superior.	Those *women's* language skills are superior.	
The *oxens* hoofs are short.	The *oxen's* hoofs are short.	*Hooves* is acceptable.
The *horse'* skin is shiny.	The *horse's* skin is shiny.	Most words that end in *s* also take *'s*, as shown in later examples.
The *mouse'* tail is long.	The *mouse's* tail is long.	
This one is for old *times's* sake.	This one is for old *times'* sake.	However, a few words that end in *s* (sound) do not take an extra *s*.
He did it for *appearances's* sake.	He did it for *appearances'* sake.	
Charles' wedding was a grand event.	*Charles's* wedding was a grand event.	Most monosyllabic or disyllabic proper names that end in *s* also take *'s*; a common mistake is to omit the *s* after the apostrophe.
Mr. *Burns'* humor is wonderful.	Mr. *Burns's* humor is wonderful.	
James' novels are serious.	*James's* novels are serious.	
Thomas' acting is superb.	*Thomas's* acting is superb.	
Keats' poetry is beautiful.	*Keats's* poetry is beautiful.	

A.1.4b. Use the Correct Forms of Possessive Nouns

Incorrect	Write Correctly
The boys's boots are here.	
The ladies's dresses are sold here.	
The mens educational status was unknown.	
The childrens language skills were not described.	
Womens professions are constantly changing.	
The horse' speed is unmatched.	
The mouse' manners are awful.	
Have one for old times's sake.	
She would not do it for appearances's sake.	
Charles' graduation party was enjoyable.	
Mr. Burns' 100th birthday celebration was cancelled.	
James' writings are philosophical.	
Thomas' lecture was boring.	
Keats' poetry is immortal.	

A.1.4a., correct forms of possessive nouns *(continued)*

Incorrect	Correct	Note
Jesus's story is moving.	*Jesus'* story is moving.	Names ending with *sus* or *ses*, that, when combined with *'s*, are awkward to pronounce, take only an apostrophe.
Moses's Ten Commandments	*Moses'* Ten Commandments	
Plato was *Socrates's* famous pupil.	Plato was *Socrates'* famous pupil.	Classical names that end with *es* also take only an apostrophe (Demosthenes', Euripides').
The *Browns's* house is large.	The *Browns'* house is large. (Correct: Browns's *shoes* are large.)	Only the apostrophe is used to form possessives in the case of plural forms of family names.
The *Thomas's* cars were stolen.	The *Thomas'* cars were stolen. (Correct: Thomas's car *was* stolen.)	

A.1.4b., correct forms of possessive nouns *(continued)*

Incorrect	Write Correctly
Jesus's kindness was boundless.	
Moses's laws are ancient.	
The dialogue was Socrates's teaching method.	
The Jones's hospitality is wonderful.	
The Thomas's vacation was cut short.	

A.1.4a., correct forms of possessive nouns *(continued)*

Incorrect	Correct	Note
We went to *Tom's* and *Jerry's* Pizza Place.	We went to *Tom* and *Jerry's* Pizza Place. *(Two owners of the place.)*	In the case of group possession, only the last name takes the *'s*.
We will take *Jim's* and *Jean's* car.	We will take *Jim* and *Jean's* car. *(Two owners of the same car.)*	
Lent's and *Bent's* book is very interesting.	*Lent* and *Bent's* book is very interesting. *(Coauthors of the same book.)*	
We will take *Linda* and *John's* cars.	We will take *Linda's* and *John's* cars. *(Independent owners of two cars.)*	In the case of separate possessions of multiple objects or characteristics, each name takes the *'s*.
Steinbeck style is different from *Saroyan's*.	*Steinbeck's* style is different from *Saroyan's*. *(Two authors, two styles.)*	
Kent book is interesting, but *Stein's* is boring.	*Kent's* book is interesting, but *Stein's* is boring. *(Two authors, two books.)*	

A.1.4b., correct forms of possessive nouns *(continued)*

Incorrect	Write Correctly
Dean's and Don's Italian restaurant is excellent. *(Two owners of the place.)*	
We borrowed Tom's and Joan's car. *(Two owners of the same car.)*	
Tent's and Nent's book on anatomy is fascinating. *(Coauthors of the same book.)*	
We will take Jim and Kim's vans. *(Independent owners of two vans.)*	
Hemingway style is different from Faulkner's. *(Two authors, two styles.)*	
Knott book has drawings, but Steel's has color pictures. *(Two authors, two books.)*	

A.1.5a. Use the Possessive Forms of Pronouns Correctly

The possessive personal pronouns *hers*, *his*, *its*, *ours*, *yours*, *theirs*, and *mine* are called *absolute* possessives, which do not take an apostrophe. Possessive forms of indefinite pronouns, on the other hand, take an apostrophe and *s* (*'s*).

Incorrect	Correct	Note
This book is *her's*.	This book is *hers*.	Do not use an apostrophe to form absolute possessive pronouns.
This hat is *his'*.	This hat is *his*.	
It's tail is long.	*Its* tail is long.	
These are *ours'*.	These are *ours*.	
Isn't she a friend of *your's*?	Isn't she a friend of *yours*?	
This is *their's*.	This is *theirs*.	
That is *mine's*.	That is *mine*.	
Anyones money will do.	*Anyone's* money will do.	Use an apostrophe and *s* (*'s*) to form possessive forms of indefinite pronouns.
Who will be next is *anybodys* guess.	Who will be next is *anybody's* guess.	
Paying taxes is *everyones* responsibility.	Paying taxes is *everyone's* responsibility.	
Someones problems are not his concern.	*Someone's* problems are not his concern.	

A.1.6a. Distinguish Contractions From Possessives

Do not confuse some contracted forms with possessives.

Incorrect	Correct	Note
They're cat is lost.	*Their* cat is lost. *They're* gone now.	*They're* is the contracted form of *they are*, and *their* is a possessive form.
You're office was closed.	*Your* office was closed. *You're* not in your office.	*You're* is the contracted form of *you are*, and *your* is a possessive form.
Who's wallet is this?	*Whose* wallet is this?	*Who's* is the contracted form of *who is*, and *whose* is the possessive form.

A.1.5b. Use the Possessive Forms of Pronouns Correctly

Incorrect	Write Correctly
Is it her's?	
I think it is his'.	
It's mouth is wide.	
Are these ours'?	
I met a friend of your's.	
It may be their's.	
Give me mine's.	
He will take anyones advice.	
He will use anybodys car.	
Taking care of the homeless is everyones responsibility.	
Those ethical concerns are someones problem.	

A.1.6b. Distinguish Contractions From Possessives

When appropriate, use the correct contracted form.

Incorrect	Write Correctly
Their in London this summer.	
Your not home tomorrow?	
They're man is not here.	
You're home is big.	
Who's side are you on?	

Unusual Singulars and Plurals

A.1.7a. Use Unusual Singulars and Plurals Correctly

- Note that in popular usage, some unusual plurals are accepted as singulars (e.g., *data is* is often seen and heard in media, but it is not accepted in scientific and professional writing).
- In scientific and professional writing, these words are used more precisely.

Incorrect	Correct	Note
Data *is* presented in Table 1.	Data *are* presented in Table 1.	*Data* is plural.
The *datum are* interesting.	The *datum is* interesting.	*Datum* is singular.
The *phenomena* of vocal abuse *is* widespread.	The *phenomenon* of vocal abuse *is* widespread.	*Phenomena* is plural.
These *phenomenon* have been recorded.	These *phenomena have* been recorded.	*Phenomenon* is singular.
There is no single *loci* of stuttering.	There is no single *locus* of stuttering.	*Locus* is singular.
The *loci* of stuttering *is* well known.	The *loci* of stuttering *are* well known.	*Loci* is plural.
The year of publication should be in *parenthesis.*	The year of publication should be in *parentheses.*	*Parentheses* is plural.
The closing *parentheses* is missing.	The closing *parenthesis* is missing.	The sentence requires the singular *parenthesis.*
I wrote a *theses.*	I wrote a *thesis.*	*Thesis* is singular.
I read *several thesis* before I selected my research topic.	I read *several theses* before I selected my research topic.	*Theses* is plural.
The participants were from the lower socioeconomic *strata.*	The participants were from the lower socioeconomic *stratum.*	*Stratum* is singular.
The participants were from *several* social *stratum.*	The participants were from *several* social *strata.*	*Strata* is plural.
The *papilloma* are benign growths.	*Papillomata* are benign growths. A *papilloma* is a benign growth.	*Papillomas* is an accepted plural form, however.
I will use a 90% correct *criteria.*	I will use a 90% correct *criterion.*	*Criterion* is singular.
I used two *criterion* of accuracy.	I used two *criteria* of accuracy.	*Criteria* is plural.
He removed *cortex* from several skulls.	He removed *cortices* from several skulls.	*Cortexes* also is an accepted plural.

Unusual Singulars and Plurals

A.1.7b. Use Unusual Singulars and Plurals Correctly

Incorrect	Write Correctly
Her data is quite complex.	
Scientists cannot control many natural phenomenon.	
The phenomena of central auditory processing is a mystery.	
The loci of vocal nodules is variable within a small range.	
Check the closing parentheses of all quotations.	
Put that statement within parenthesis.	
I found no support for that theses.	
All of our thesis are in the library.	
Study participants should be drawn from at least three social stratum.	
The papillomata is a benign growth.	

A.1.7a., use unusual singulars and plurals correctly *(continued)*

Incorrect	Correct	Note
I found several scholarly *corpus* on the subject.	I found several scholarly *corpora* on the subject.	*Corpora* is plural.
The book has seven *appendix.*	The book has seven *appendixes.*	The APA *Manual* recommends *appendixes*; some other authorities recommend *appendices.*
The author and subject *index* are helpful.	The author and subject *indexes* are helpful.	The APA *Manual* recommends *indexes*; some other authorities recommend *indices.*
I have *several basis* for my argument.	I have *several bases* for my argument.	*Bases* is plural.
I had *many crisis.*	I had *many crises.*	*Crises* is plural.
The term *nucleus* refers to central *cores* of structures.	The term *nuclei* refers to central *cores* of structures.	*Nuclei* is the plural form of nucleus.

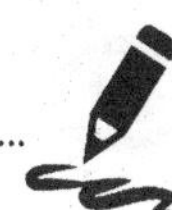

A.1.7b., use unusual singulars and plurals correctly *(continued)*

Incorrect	Write Correctly
Her grading criteria for an A is 90%.	
Good grades and high GRE scores are two criterion for admission.	
Lesion in a single cortices does not prove anything.	
Corpora means a single collection of scholarly writings.	
I found too many appendix in the book.	
He did not have a single bases for his statement.	
I can handle one crises in a semester.	
The term *nuclei* means a central core of structures.	

Comma

A.1.8a. Use a Serial Comma

A serial comma separates parallel terms in a series. In the term *women, men, and children*, the second comma before *and* is a serial comma. When you use three or more terms connected with a single conjunction, use a comma after each term that precedes the conjunction. Note that the print media may not use a serial comma.

<table>
<tr><th>Incorrect</th><th>Correct</th><th>Note</th></tr>
<tr><td>The child had misarticulations, delayed language and hearing loss.</td><td>The child had misarticulations, delayed language, and hearing loss.</td><td rowspan="2">Serial comma before the conjunction and.</td></tr>
<tr><td>Our clinicians are intelligent, compassionate and competent.</td><td>Our clinicians are intelligent, compassionate, and competent.</td></tr>
<tr><td>Each token may be exchanged for a sticker, a piece of gum or a small toy.</td><td>Each token may be exchanged for a sticker, a piece of gum, or a small toy.</td><td rowspan="2">Serial comma before the conjunction or.</td></tr>
<tr><td>Age, education, health, occupation or gender may be a significant variable in this study.</td><td>Age, education, health, occupation, or gender may be a significant variable in this study.</td></tr>
</table>

A.1.9a. Do Not Use a Serial Comma When You Write Only Two Parallel Terms and Connect Them With a Conjunction

<table>
<tr><th>Incorrect</th><th>Correct</th><th>Note</th></tr>
<tr><td>The person with aphasia had naming, and echolalia.</td><td>The person with aphasia had naming and echolalia.</td><td rowspan="4">In each case, only two terms are joined by a different conjunction (and, or).</td></tr>
<tr><td>I will recruit both male, and female participants.</td><td>I will recruit both male and female participants.</td></tr>
<tr><td>Plastic tokens, or stickers will be the reinforcers.</td><td>Plastic tokens or stickers will be the reinforcers.</td></tr>
<tr><td>The study revealed that age, or severity predicts improvement.</td><td>The study revealed that age or severity predicts improvement.</td></tr>
</table>

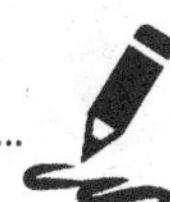

Comma

A1.8b. Use a Serial Comma

Incorrect	Write Correctly
I will teach the plural morpheme, the auxiliary and the copula.	
Sensory, neural and sensorineural hearing losses must be distinguished.	
The clients may choose counseling, syllable prolongation, time-out or response cost as treatment.	
Verbal praise, smiles or tokens will be reinforcers.	

A.1.9b. Do Not Use a Serial Comma When You Write Only Two Parallel Terms and Connect Them With a Conjunction

Incorrect	Write Correctly
We noticed omissions, and distortions of speech sounds.	
Assessment revealed a large tongue, and missing canine teeth.	
Treatment may start at the word, or the phrase level.	
The client can select an analog, or digital hearing aid.	

A.1.10a. Use a Comma to Separate Parenthetic Expressions That Are Not in Parentheses

Parenthetic expressions interject an additional idea into a sentence.

Incorrect	Correct
The woman who stuttered though she could not remember it had received treatment before.	The woman who stuttered, though she could not remember it, had received treatment before.
The client who was extremely dysfluent hesitated before starting to read aloud.	The client, who was extremely dysfluent, hesitated before starting to read aloud.
The woman a professional wrestler in her 50s had a stroke.	The woman, a professional wrestler in her 50s, had a stroke.
The mean length of utterance when calculated properly can be a good index of early language development.	The mean length of utterance, when calculated properly, can be a good index of early language development.

A.1.11a. Place a Comma Before a Conjunction Introducing an Independent Clause

An independent clause can stand alone as a sentence; the terms after the conjunction in the correct example form an independent clause.

Incorrect	Correct
I suggested a treatment program but the client was disinterested.	I suggested a treatment program, but the client was disinterested.
The man was diagnosed with aphasia and the prognosis for recovery was poor.	The man was diagnosed with aphasia, and the prognosis for recovery was poor.
Standardized tests should be administered properly or they will yield meaningless scores.	Standardized tests should be administered properly, or they will yield meaningless scores.

A.1.12a. Do Not Use a Comma Before a Conjunction That Is Followed by a Dependent Clause

A dependent clause (like the one shown in the correct example starting with a conjunction) cannot stand alone.

Incorrect	Correct
The child was first assessed for speech and language, and then was referred to the psychologist.	The child was first assessed for speech and language and then was referred to the psychologist.
A treatment plan was developed, and later it was implemented.	A treatment plan was developed and later it was implemented.

A.1.10b. Use a Comma to Separate Parenthetic Expressions That Are Not in Parentheses

Incorrect	Write Correctly
The child with misarticulations even though capable did not do well.	
The client who had aphasia could not readily name the objects shown.	

A.1.11b. Place a Comma Before a Conjunction Introducing an Independent Clause

Incorrect	Write Correctly
The client's mother was asked to attend the sessions but her attendance was poor.	
The students were asked to make oral presentations but they were reluctant.	
The teacher cooperated with the clinician and the children benefited.	
The father conducted treatment sessions at home and the progress was excellent.	

A.1.12b. Do Not Use a Comma Before a Conjunction That Is Followed by a Dependent Clause

Incorrect	Write Correctly
The client was treated first, and then was offered a follow-up assessment.	
Several goals were established, and will be discussed with the parents.	

Dash

A.1.13a. Prefer an Em Dash to a Comma to Set Off an Abrupt Break

Note: On a computer, if you type two dashes (--) with no space in between or on either side of the dashes, they will be converted to an *em dash* (printed as an unbroken line).

Not Preferred	Preferred
The speech discrimination test, a part of audiological evaluation, revealed no problems.	The speech discrimination test—a part of audiological evaluation—revealed no problems.
The administration of a pure probe, if it is administered at all, requires much prior work.	The administration of a pure probe—if it is administered at all—requires much prior work.

Note: No space separates the dashes (or *em dashes*) and the word that precedes or follows them.

Semicolon

A.1.14a. Join Independent Clauses With a Semicolon When the Clauses Are Not Joined by a Conjunction

The two independent clauses may be rewritten as two separate sentences.

Incorrect	Correct
Stuttering is a speech problem, it should not be ignored.	Stuttering is a speech problem; it should not be ignored. Stuttering is a speech problem. It should not be ignored.
Dysphagia may cause serious concerns, it can be life-threatening.	Dysphagia may cause serious concerns; it can be life-threatening. Dysphagia may cause serious concerns. It can be life-threatening.
Language disorders can lead to poor academic performance, they should be promptly treated.	Language disorders can lead to poor academic performance; they should be promptly treated. Language disorders can lead to poor academic performance. They should be promptly treated.

Dash

A.1.13b. Prefer an Em Dash to a Comma to Set Off an Abrupt Break

Not Preferred	Preferred
Modeling, a basic treatment procedure, will be used when the client fails to imitate.	
Treatment of stuttering, unless the clinician believes in spontaneous recovery, should be started as early as possible.	
The incidence of noise-induced hearing loss, a hazardous but controllable by-product of civilization, is on the increase.	

Semicolon

A.1.14b. Use a Semicolon to Join Independent Clauses That Are Not Joined by a Conjunction

Alternatively, write them as two separate sentences.

Incorrect	Write Correctly
Dementia is a progressive disorder, it often is undetected in its early stages.	1. 2.
Early treatment of stuttering is effective, this is unknown to some clinicians.	1. 2.
Speech disorders may persist in some children, they should be promptly treated.	1. 2.
Language acquisition is an interesting subject, I might do a thesis on it.	1. 2.

Agreement

A.1.15a. Follow the Rules of Agreement

- Subject and verb should agree in number.
- The terms that intervene between the noun phrase and the verb do not affect agreement.

Take note of exceptions:

- The pronouns *they*, *them*, *their*, and *themselves* that are technically plurals are used as generic third-person singular pronouns to refer to a person whose gender is unknown, irrelevant, unspecified, or known to be nonbinary:
  - A responsible *student* knows that *they* should study hard.
  - *Everyone* in the camp got a gift delivered to *them.*
  - Each *individual* is responsible for *their* actions.
  - *A therapist* should continuously update *themselves.* [The term *themself* is also acceptable, but *themselves* is more common.]

Incorrect	Correct	Note
No single dysfluency *type*—prolongations or sound repetitions—*justify* diagnosis.	No single dysfluency *type*—prolongations or sound repetitions—*justifies* diagnosis.	No single dysfluency *type justifies* diagnosis.
She is one of *those* clinicians who *is* always prepared for *her* sessions.	She is one of *those* clinicians who *are* always prepared for *their* sessions.	*clinicians* who *are* always prepared for their sessions
These *techniques*, when used correctly, *is* known to be effective.	These *techniques*, when used correctly, *are* known to be effective.	*Techniques are* known to be effective.

Agreement

A.1.15b. Follow the Rules of Agreement

Incorrect	Write Correctly
A speech disorder—whether it contains a few or many misarticulations—indicate a need for treatment.	
Naming problems, along with agrammatism, characterizes aphasia.	
He is one of those individuals who is always late.	
Tokens, when dispensed for a correct response, increases the rate of progress.	

A.1.15a., follow the rules of agreement *(continued)*

Incorrect	Correct	Note
Error *scores,* along with the correct score, *was* analyzed.	Error *scores,* along with the correct score, *were* analyzed.	Error *scores were* analyzed.
Every child and adult *go* through the same procedure.	*Every* child and adult *goes* through the same procedure.	A singular verb is used when *every* or *each* precedes a compound subject joined by *and.*
Each man and woman *consider* whether it is right.	*Each* man and woman *considers* whether it is right.	
Either verbal praise *or* informative feedback *are* combined with modeling.	*Either* verbal praise *or* informative feedback *is* combined with modeling.	When two subjects are linked by *or, either/or,* or *neither/nor,* the verb must be plural if both the subjects are plural and singular if both the subjects are singular.
Either words *or* morphemes *is* appropriate for calculating MLUs.	*Either* words *or* morphemes *are* appropriate for calculating MLUs.	
Neither he *nor* she *were* interested in the proposal.	*Neither* he *nor* she *was* interested in the proposal.	
Neither the stimuli *nor* the reinforcers *was* effective.	*Neither* the stimuli *nor* the reinforcers *were* effective.	
Neither the treatments *nor* the result *are* replicable.	*Neither* the treatments *nor* the result *is* replicable.	When a singular and a plural subject are linked by *neither/nor, either/or,* or *not only/but also,* the verb form is determined by the subject that is nearer to it.
Either the tokens *or* the verbal praise *are* appropriate.	*Either* the tokens or the verbal praise *is* appropriate.	
Not only the treatment, *but also* the *settings, tends* to affect the outcome.	*Not only* the treatment *but also* the *settings tend* to affect the outcome.	

A.1.15b., follow the rules of agreement *(continued)*

Incorrect	Write Correctly
Every client and a family member receive training in treatment.	
Either time-out or response cost for incorrect responses are combined with positive reinforcement.	
Neither the procedure nor the outcome were clear.	
Neither the client nor his parents was cooperative.	
Neither stutterings nor the phonological processes is easily measured.	
Either verbal feedback or tokens is given to the client for her correct responses.	
Not only the client, but also his colleagues, tends to accept the suggestion.	
Percentage of dysfluency rates, along with the frequency of each dysfluency, is presented in Table 1.	
Either verbal feedback or tokens is given to the client for her correct responses.	
Either family support or teacher support are essential for maintenance of treatment effects.	
Neither the parents nor the grandparents was cooperative.	
Not only the rate of speech, but also the syllable prolongations, affects fluency.	

A.1.15a., follow the rules of agreement *(continued)*

Incorrect	Correct	Note
Mother *and* child was interviewed together.	Mother *and* child were interviewed together.	Compound subjects joined by *and* have plural verbs.
Who says *country and western* are dead?	Who says *country and western* is dead?	Expressions containing *and* that suggest a single concept (e.g., *country and western*) use singular verbs.
Both of us *is* busy.	*Both* of us *are* busy.	A few indefinite pronouns (*both, many, several, few, others*) are always plural and take plural verbs.
Either of them *are* acceptable.	*Either* of them *is* acceptable.	Most other indefinite pronouns (*another, anyone, everyone, each, either, neither, anything, everything, something*, and *somebody*) are singular and take singular verbs.
Some of *this* effect *are* understandable.	Some of *this* effect *is* understandable.	Some indefinite pronouns (*some, all, none, any, more*, and *most*) can be singular or plural. The verb form is singular or plural depending on the noun the pronoun refers to.
Some of *these* effects *is* understandable.	Some of *these* effects *are* understandable.	
The *group were* tested in a single session.	The *group was* tested in a single session.	Collective nouns can take singular verbs (if they refer to a single unit) or plural verbs (if they refer to individuals or elements of that unit).
Seven *individuals* in the group *was* retested.	Seven *individuals* in the group *were* retested.	
The *majority were* against the idea. A *majority* of people *was* against the idea.	The *majority was* against the idea. A *majority* of people *were* against the idea.	*The majority* is singular; *a majority of people* is plural.

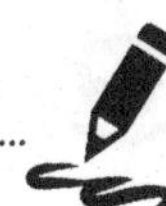

A.1.15b., follow the rules of agreement *(continued)*

Incorrect	Write Correctly
The experimental group were treated.	
Four participants in the control group was dropped from the study.	
The clinician and the client's sister was in the same treatment room.	
Who says rock 'n' roll are only for the older people?	
Both of us is willing to do it.	
Several of the group is unhappy.	
Some of this mess are your responsibility.	
Some of these effects is unexplained.	
The majority were unimpressed.	
A majority of clinicians tends to agree.	

A.1.15a., follow the rules of agreement *(continued)*

Incorrect	Correct	Note
The *news are* bad.	The *news is* bad.	Some words that are typically in the plural form still take singular verbs.
Statistics are an exciting field.	*Statistics is* an exciting field.	
Economics are an inexact science.	*Economics is* an inexact science.	
Statistics shows that the county poverty rate is high.	*Statistics show* that the county poverty rate is high.	When *statistics* refers to numbers, it takes a plural verb.
A hurricane *is* a terrifying *phenomena.*	A hurricane *is* a terrifying *phenomenon.*	*Phenomenon* is singular, and *phenomena* is plural.
They offered *many thesis*, but none too exciting.	They offered *many theses*, but none too exciting.	*Theses* is plural, and *thesis* is singular.
His *data was* unconvincing.	His *data were* unconvincing.	In the APA style of scientific writing, the term *data* is plural, and *datum* is singular. Journalists who follow the Associated Press style guide use *data* as singular.

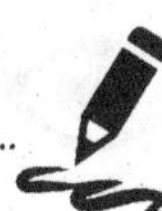

A.1.15b., follow the rules of agreement *(continued)*

Incorrect	Write Correctly
The local news tend to focus on crime.	
Statistics suggests fewer problems.	
Statistics are one of the two courses.	
Politics are full of scoundrels.	
The phenomenon of earthquakes are poorly understood.	
It is a scary natural phenomena.	
My theses is as good as yours.	
The theses explaining language learning does not interest me.	
His data is a bit confusing.	
The datum are enlightening.	

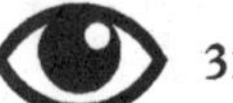

Modifiers

A.1.16a. Use Modifiers Correctly

To avoid confusion in the use of modifiers, keep the related words together.

<table>
<tr><th>Incorrect</th><th>Correct</th><th>Note</th></tr>
<tr><td>The author and her assistants tested the hearing of all participants using the procedure described earlier.</td><td>The author and her assistants, using the procedure described earlier, tested the hearing of all participants.</td><td>Who used the procedure? Not the participants!</td></tr>
<tr><td>Distant and mysterious, he stared at the sky.</td><td>He stared at the distant and mysterious sky.</td><td>Who was mysterious and distant? Not he!</td></tr>
<tr><td>Several additional effects are observed using this technique in clients.</td><td>Several additional effects are observed in clients using this technique.</td><td>Who observed effects in whom?</td></tr>
<tr><td>Using the procedure, the participants were screened for hearing problems by the experimenter.</td><td>Using the procedure, the experimenter screened the participants for hearing problems.</td><td>Who used the procedure?</td></tr>
<tr><td>The study merely provided a partial support for the hypothesis.</td><td>The study provided merely a partial support for the hypothesis.</td><td rowspan="3">Place the following modifiers immediately before the words they modify: almost, only, even, hardly, merely, nearly, exactly, scarcely, just, and simply.</td></tr>
<tr><td>Teaching skills without concern for maintenance is hardly sufficient.</td><td>It is hardly sufficient to teach skills without concern for maintenance.</td></tr>
<tr><td>Simply sampling language just once is not sufficient.</td><td>It simply is not sufficient to sample language just once.</td></tr>
<tr><td>Several problems have been observed using negative reinforcement.</td><td>Several problems have been observed when clinicians used negative reinforcement.</td><td>Using negative reinforcement is a dangling modifier because it has no head word.</td></tr>
</table>

Modifiers

A.1.16b. Use Modifiers Correctly

Incorrect	Write Correctly
The clinician treated stuttering persons using the syllable stretching procedure.	
Consistent with other studies, Smith and Smith (1993) found that cochlear implants are beneficial. *Hint:* What were consistent? Results or the authors?	
Using the Utah Test, the children's language was screened by the experimenter.	
The treatment only was partially effective.	
He said he was leaving, in a thundering voice.	
The client only had three tokens. (The client had nothing other than three tokens.)	Rewrite the sentence to mean that the client had *no more than* three tokens.
Using tokens, the child was reinforced.	Rewrite to include a person who reinforced the child.
To get a better grade, a long paper was written.	Rewrite the sentence in the active voice and include a subject (e.g., a person's name).
The lecture was made interesting by including videos and computer programs.	Rewrite in the active voice and include a subject.

Pronouns

- Pronouns, which replace nouns, should clarify what they replace.
- The nouns that pronouns replace are called *antecedents.*
- Pronouns should agree with the replaced noun's (antecedent's) number and gender.

A.1.17a. Clarify the Referents of Pronouns

Incorrect	Correct	Note
I will use toys and pictures as stimuli and give reinforcers for correct responses. *They* will be used continuously.	I will use toys and pictures as stimuli and give reinforcers for correct responses. *These reinforcers* will be used continuously.	*They* refers to what? Correct responses or reinforcers?
A lesion in Broca's area, in the left frontal cortex, causes Broca's aphasia. *It* may be diagnosed only after careful examination.	A lesion in Broca's area, in the left frontal cortex, may be diagnosed only after careful examination. *Such a lesion* causes Broca's aphasia.	*What* may be diagnosed? The corrected statement says it is the lesion.
Mark went with John because he did not know the address.	Mark did not know the address, so he went with John.	*Who* did not know the address?
The client told the clinician that she was happy.	The client told the clinician, "I am happy."	*Who* was happy?

A.1.18a. Let the Pronoun Agree in Number With Its Antecedent

See A.1.15a., Follow the Rules of Agreement, for related examples of correct and incorrect agreement.

Incorrect	Correct	Note
Clinicians may not recognize that her own limitations affect treatment outcomes.	Clinicians may not recognize that their own limitations affect treatment outcomes.	The plural (clinicians) did not agree with the singular pronoun (*her*).
Neither the children who stuttered nor the children who spoke with typical fluency let his or her test performance suffer.	Neither the children who stuttered nor the children who spoke with typical fluency let their test performance suffer.	Plural nouns (children) paired with *their.*

A.1.19a. Use the Proper Case of Pronoun

<table>
<tr><th>Incorrect</th><th>Correct</th><th>Note</th></tr>
<tr><td>Between you and I.</td><td>Between you and me.</td><td></td></tr>
<tr><td>They have invited you and myself.</td><td>They have invited you and me.</td><td rowspan="2">Possessive pronouns hers, theirs, ours, and its do not take the apostrophe.</td></tr>
<tr><td>Her's is the big house.</td><td>Hers is the big house.</td></tr>
</table>

Pronouns

A.1.17b. Clarify the Referents of Pronouns

Incorrect	Write Correctly
We use stimuli, modeling, and positive feedback. It will be used only when the child does not imitate, however.	
Many studies, conducted by several investigators, have confirmed this. They indicate that we should program maintenance.	
The clinician went with the supervisor because she did not know the practicum site.	
Jane told her female boss that she was upset.	

A.1.18b. Let the Pronoun Agree in Number With Its Antecedent

Incorrect	Correct
Even if the clinicians are pleased, clients may not be pleased with his or her own success in treatment.	
Men with aphasia may report that he could not recall the names.	
Neither the clinicians nor the parents sought expressed his or her disappointment.	

A.1.19b. Use the Proper Case of Pronoun

Incorrect	Write Correctly
You and myself should complete the assessment.	
He told Tom and I to finish the job.	
Ours' is an old house.	

Sentence Fragments

A.1.20a. Do Not Break a Single Sentence Into Two Parts

Incorrect	Correct
Upon subjective evaluation. The client's voice was judged normal.	Upon subjective evaluation, the client's voice was judged normal.
The man finally agreed to be tested. After much coaxing from his wife.	After much coaxing from his wife, the man finally agreed to be tested.
I work with 10 children. All with speech sound disorders.	I work with 10 children, all with speech sound disorders.
Children with hearing loss have delayed oral language. And also may have voice problems.	Many children with hearing loss have delayed oral language and also may have voice problems.
I will select 20 participants for the experiment. Based on the selection criteria.	Based on the selection criteria, I will select 20 participants.
My client with dysphagia is improving. Because of the treatment.	Because of the treatment, my client with dysphagia is improving.

A.1.21a. Do Not Write Sentence Fragments as a Series of Declarative Statements

Incorrect	Correct
Graduate students have many problems. Lack of money. Family responsibilities. Job stress.	Graduate students have many problems, including lack of money, family responsibilities, and job stress.
Clinicians should consider several factors in planning therapy sessions. Like stimulus materials. Reinforcers to be given. Criteria for learning.	Clinicians should consider several factors in planning therapy sessions. For instance, stimulus materials to be used, reinforcers to be given, and criteria for learning should be considered before therapy.

A.1.22a. Do Not Punctuate Appositives

Incorrect	Correct
Several authorities have advocated this type of therapy. For example, van Riper (1971) and Johnson (1958).	Several authorities have advocated this type of therapy, including van Riper (1971) and Johnson (1958).
Several theories have suggested that poor self-image causes language delay in children. For instance, the self-image-is-king theory and the sharper image theory.	Several theories—for example, the self-image-is-king theory and the sharper image theory—have suggested that poor self-image causes language delay in children.

Sentence Fragments

A.1.20b. Do Not Break a Single Sentence Into Two Parts

Incorrect	Write Correctly
I will treat 12 children with language disorders. Divided into two groups.	
The child finally began to cooperate. After two sessions of crying.	
I tested the hearing of all participants. In a sound-treated room.	
The client made excellent progress. In the final four sessions.	
Three phonological processes were eliminated. All during this semester.	

A.1.21b. Do Not Write Sentence Fragments as a Series of Declarative Statements

Incorrect	Correct
Big cities offer many advantages. Green parks. Sports arenas. Music concerts.	
School clinicians face several challenges. Like uncooperative parents. Paperwork. Pressure from administrators.	

A.1.22b. Do Not Punctuate Appositives

Incorrect	Correct
Several studies have recommended this procedure. For example, those by Bloodstein (1971) and Thompson (2015).	
There are several genetic theories of stuttering. For instance, the multifactor theory and recessive gene theory.	

Nouns and Adjectives

A.1.23a. Use Certain Terms Only in Their Adjectival Forms

Incorrect	Correct	Note
The *paraplegic* also has aphasia.	The *person with paraplegia* also has aphasia.	The incorrect versions put the disability first, not the person. The terms in italics within the incorrect constructions are used as nouns, which are preferably used only as adjectives. Some families and disability advocates suggest that *autistic* is an acceptable noun because it is a claimed identity (like the Deaf).
The *aphasic* has naming problems.	The *man with aphasia* has naming problems.	
The *autistic* has echolalia.	The *child with autism* has echolalia.	
Ten stutterers will be selected.	Ten *persons with stuttering* will be selected.	

A.1.24a. Do Not Turn a Noun Into a Verb

Although many "verbized" nouns are popular and become established over time, a careful writer will be more cautious in using what seems to be acceptable.

Incorrect	Correct	Note
We will *agendize* this matter for the next meeting.	We will place this matter on the next meeting's agenda.	The popular tendency to *ize* a noun has created many awkward verbs.
ASHA should not be *factionalized.*	ASHA should not be factious.	
The APA *Manual* has a *rigidized* format for empirical articles.	The APA *Manual* has a rigid format for empirical articles.	
Many clinicians have *therapized* Mr. Wilson who stutters.	Many clinicians have treated Mr. Wilson who stutters.	
Women and minority groups should never be *inferiorized.*	No one should think that women and minority groups are inferior.	
First, I *baselined* the target behaviors.	First, I established baselines of the target behaviors. *or* First, I baserated the target behaviors.	Note that the word *baserate* may be used both as a noun and as a verb (e.g., *baserates* or *baserated*).
He finally *verbalized* his secret intentions.	He finally revealed his secret intentions. *or* He finally spoke about his secret intentions.	Even though the term *verbalize* is often used, the alternatives are more direct and simpler.

Nouns and Adjectives

A.1.23b. Use Certain Terms Only in Their Adjectival Forms

Incorrect	Write Correctly
The dysarthric has multiple communication disorders.	
The retarded's language is delayed.	*Hint:* Intellectual disabilities
The hemiplegic has motor speech disorders.	
Many apraxics exhibit articulatory groping problems.	
The autistic fails to develop emotional attachment.	

A.1.24b. Do Not Turn a Noun Into a Verb

Incorrect	Write Correctly
She guested on a TV show.	
It is necessary to baseline behaviors before starting treatment.	
He thefted my textbooks.	
We partnershipped with the community.	
Our purpose is now collectivized.	
The heroes who died in the war will be funeralized in a state ceremony.	

Participial Phrase

A.1.25a. Let a Participial Phrase at the Beginning of a Sentence Refer to the Grammatical Subject

A participle is a verbal phrase that can function as an adjective; for example, "*Dropped from the second floor*, the ball bounced around" contains the italicized participial phrase. This verbal phrase, acting as an adjective, refers to *the ball*, the subject of the sentence. When the participial phrase does not refer to the grammatical subject in the sentence, it may be described as *dangling* and sound ludicrous: "*Dropped from the second floor*, I saw the ball bounce around." In this dangling participial phrase, the person, not the ball, is dropped from the second floor!

Incorrect	Correct	Note
A clinician of *great reputation*, I asked her to treat the client.	A clinician of great reputation, *she* was asked to treat the client.	Who was of great reputation?
On discussing treatment options with the client's family, they responded favorably to the clinician.	On discussing treatment options with the client's family, *the clinician* received favorable responses.	Who discussed and who responded favorably are not clear in the incorrect version.
Being in a fixer-upper condition, I found the house a good bargain.	Being in a fixer-upper condition, the house was a good bargain.	The house, not the speaker, was in a fixer-upper condition.
Critically evaluating the evidence presented, the article provides good insight into language acquisition.	*Critically evaluating the evidence presented*, I found the article to provide good insight into language acquisition.	The reader, not the article, critically evaluated the evidence presented.

Participial Phrase

A.1.25b. Let a Participial Phrase at the Beginning of a Sentence Refer to the Grammatical Subject

Incorrect	Write Correctly
Inexperienced in the treatment of dysphagia, the treatment goals were thought to be easy to establish.	*Hint:* Who was inexperienced?
Without a friend to study with, the failure was inevitable.	*Hint:* Whose failure?
Without help from parents, maintenance of target behaviors was difficult.	*Hint:* Whose maintenance?
Studying carefully the data presented, the article makes a good contribution to treatment research.	*Hint:* Who studied the data carefully?

A.2. Basic Rules of Composition

Structure of Research Papers

A.2.1a. Design a Broad Outline of Your Paper

- Before beginning to write a paper or an essay, make a broad outline of it.
- Write down the major topics you want to address in the paper.
- Type each major topic as a Level 1 heading.
- Make some preliminary notes under each of the major topics to be addressed.

Theories of Language Acquisition

Brigitte Lopez

Brief Historical Introduction to the Study of Language (*untitled*)

(The ancient and modern study of language, involvement of different disciplines, and so forth)

Linguistic Theories of Language Acquisition

(Descriptive linguistics, transformational generative grammar, neurolinguistic theories, and so forth)

Psychological Theories of Language Acquisition

(Behavioral explanations, cognitive explanations, incidental learning, statistical learning, infant-directed speech, interactive explanations, and so forth)

Recent Developments in Theoretical Explanations

(Integration of different views, suggestions from cross-cultural studies)

Critical Evaluation of Theories

(most are deductive-speculative; lack experimental support)

Summary and Conclusions

(Need for additional research, future directions)

Note: There is no one correct outline for a topic. The first outline usually is modified.

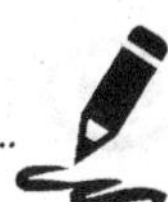

Structure of Research Papers

A.2.1b. Design a Broad Outline of Your Paper

Select a major academic or clinical topic and design an outline for it. Use the Level 1 heading style shown in A.2.1a. Show your notes.

A.2.2a. Design Headings and Subheadings of Your Paper

- Select levels of headings; see B.3.7 for examples.
- Use the major headings of your initial outline.
- Give technical headings.
- Prefer the shorter headings to the longer headings.
- Use those headings in your paper.
- Keep the number of subheadings under major headings roughly similar.
- Write at least two paragraphs under each heading or subheading.

Theories of Language Acquisition

Brigette Lopez

Brief Historical Introduction to the Study of Language (*untitled*)

Linguistic Theories of Language Acquisition

Descriptive Linguistic Theories Transformational Generative Theories Generative Semantic Theories

Neurolinguistic Theories

Recent Linguistic Developments

Psychological Theories of Language Acquisition

Behavioral Theories

Cognitive Theories

Incidental learning

Statistical learning

Infant-directed speech

Interactional Theories

Recent Developments in Theoretical Explanations

Attempts at Integrating Different Views Suggestions from Cross-Cultural Studies

Newer Theories

Critical Evaluation of Theories

Common Research Methods

Comparative Evaluation of Evidence Suggestions for Future Research

Summary and Conclusions

References

Note: The example contains only two levels of headings; you may need additional headings (see B.3.7.).

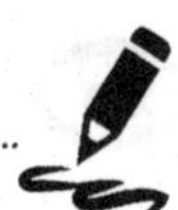

A.2.2b. Design Headings and Subheadings of Your Paper

For the outline you prepared under A.2.1b., design headings and subheadings. Revise your headings and subheadings until you can begin writing.

Composing Paragraphs

A.2.3a. Write Paragraphs That Express Related Ideas

- Express *related* ideas in a paragraph.
- Make each paragraph a conceptual unit.
- Do not mix different kinds of information in a paragraph.

Incorrect	Correct	Note
The participants will be 25 children with hearing loss. They will come from middle-class families. The children will be selected from a single school within the local school district. The school will be selected randomly. The parents of the children will have normal hearing. The intelligence of the children will be within normal limits.	The participants will be 25 children with hearing loss. They will come from middle-class families. The intelligence of the children will be within normal limits. The parents of the children will have normal hearing. The children will be selected from a single school within the local school district. The school will be selected randomly.	The incorrect version mixes up participant characteristics and their selection procedure. The correct version describes them in two paragraphs.
The client will be seen two times a week in 30-minute sessions. The initial target behaviors will be the correct production of five phonemes. In the beginning, the client will be trained on discrete trials. Later, conversational speech will be used to stabilize the production of target phonemes. The parents will be trained to help maintain the production of target phonemes. The initial training procedure will include discrete trials. A picture will be used to evoke the target phonemes in words.	The client will be seen two times a week in 30-minute sessions. The initial target behaviors will be the correct production of five phonemes. The initial training procedure will include discrete trials. A picture will be used to evoke the target phonemes in words. In the final stage of treatment, conversational speech will be used to stabilize the production of target phonemes. The parents will be trained to help maintain the production of target phonemes.	The first paragraph of the correct version describes the target behaviors. The second paragraph is about the treatment procedure. The third is about the final stage of treatment and parent training. These ideas are mixed up in the incorrect version.

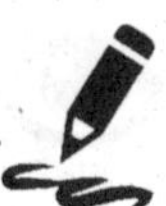

Composing Paragraphs

A.2.3b. Write Paragraphs That Express Related Ideas

Incorrect	Write Correctly
Mr. Garcia reported that he began to notice hearing problems some 5 months ago. His wife agreed that it was about that time that her husband began to turn up the volume of their television. He has always enjoyed good physical health. He has been socially active since his retirement 2 years ago. Around that time, he began to complain that his wife mumbles her speech. Mr. Garcia is a 65-year-old retired electrician. Reportedly, his hearing problem has worsened during the last several months.	

Write a Mixed-up Paragraph	Rewrite It Correctly

A.2.4a. Do Not Write Paragraphs That Are Too Long

- Break longer paragraphs into shorter ones.
- Make sure each paragraph is about related ideas.

Too Long	About Right	Note
Assessment of Timmy's speech and language will include an orofacial examination, a hearing screening, and administration of the Thompson Vocabulary Test (Thompson, 2022), the Jenson Test of Articulatory Performance (Jenson, 2019), and the Shanks Test of Syntactic Constructions (Shanks, 2023). In addition, an extended conversational speech sample will be recorded. The results of this assessment will be integrated with information obtained through case history, reports from other specialists, and information gathered through an interview of Timmy's parents. Timmy's performance on the selected standardized tests will be analyzed according to the test manuals. The conversational speech samples will be analyzed for speech and language skills. The number of correct productions of phonemes, syntactic structures, and conversational skills will be determined. Also, the mean length of utterance will be calculated using the Brown method.	Assessment of Timmy's speech and language behaviors will include an orofacial examination, a hearing screening, and administration of the Thompson Vocabulary Test (Thompson, 2012), the Jenson Test of Articulatory Performance (Jenson, 2016), and the Shanks Test of Syntactic Constructions (Shanks, 2017). In addition, an extended conversational speech sample will be recorded. The results of this assessment will be integrated with information obtained through case history, reports from other specialists, and information gathered through an interview of Timmy's parents. Timmy's performance on the selected standardized tests will be analyzed according to the test manuals. The conversational speech samples will be analyzed for speech and language skills. The number of correct productions of phonemes, syntactic structures, and conversational skills will be determined. Also, the mean length of utterance will be calculated using the Brown method.	The long paragraph of different pieces of information has been broken into smaller ones, each expressing a set of related ideas.

Note: Standardized tests should be referenced; the given examples are fictitious.

A.2.4b. Do Not Write Paragraphs That Are Too Long

Too Long	Rewrite to Make It About Right
Aural rehabilitation is an extended process in which a person with hearing loss is helped to make the best use of their residual hearing. The process begins with hearing testing, but it does not end with it. The process does not end even with a prescription for, or fitting of, a hearing aid. The purchase of a hearing aid is the beginning of aural rehabilitation. The client should be first familiarized with the workings of the hearing aid. The client should learn to change the battery, turn on the aid, adjust the volume, and so forth. The person who purchases a hearing aid should know how to take care of it, clean it periodically, and protect it from shock and other hazards. The person also should know when to take it for service. Even more important, the person with hearing loss should know how to benefit from the aid. Initially, the hearing aid's amplification of sound and noise may irritate the person or cause discomfort. A person with hearing loss may get headaches until getting used to the aid's amplified sound. The client should know how to handle the incoming, amplified signal. The audiologist helps the client recognize the meaning of sounds previously missed but now heard.	

A.2.5a. Do Not Write One-Sentence Paragraphs

- This rule applies to scientific and academic writing but not to clinical reports.
- Under the inappropriate heading, notice two single-sentence paragraphs.

Inappropriate	Appropriate	Note
The effects of communication disorders are several. The disorders create many social and occupational difficulties. Some people with communication disorders may withdraw from normal social interactions. Some employers may be unwilling to hire people with such problems. People who have communication disorders may experience certain emotional problems. Such people may be frustrated in their attempts at communication. People who stutter or those who have aphasia experience frustration when they cannot express themselves promptly.	The effects of communication disorders are several. The disorders create many social and occupational difficulties. Some people with communication disorders may withdraw from normal social interactions. Some employers may be unwilling to hire people with such problems. People with communication disorders may experience certain emotional problems. For example, people who stutter or those who have aphasia may experience frustration when they cannot express themselves promptly.	Two one-sentence paragraphs stand alone with nothing to connect them. Note that when two paragraphs are combined, wording may need to be changed to provide transition.

A.2.5b. Do Not Write One-Sentence Paragraphs

Choose an academic topic.

Write Four One-Sentence Paragraphs	Integrate the Four One-Sentence Paragraphs Into a Single Paragraph

A.2.6a. Begin and End Most Paragraphs With Transitionary Sentences

Lack of transition breaks the flow of thought and confuses the reader. To achieve smooth transition, **do** one or more of the following:

- End and begin adjacent paragraphs with a related idea.
- Suggest what will be said in the next paragraph.
- Refer to what was said in the previous paragraph.

However, **do not**

- Introduce new topics abruptly.
- Randomly shift topics across paragraphs.

Rough Transition	Smoother Transition	Note
Methods of analysis of speech sound errors have undergone many changes. Traditionally, the clinicians have made the sound-by-sound analysis to judge the accuracy of individual sound productions. In the place-voice-manner analysis, sounds are classified into patterns based on these phonetic features. Errors also are similarly classified. Phonological processes are simplifications of speech sound productions that help classify multiple errors into groups or patterns. Another approach is that of distinctive feature analysis, which was suggested before the phonological process approach.	Methods of analysis of speech sound errors have changed over the years. Traditionally, the clinicians have made the sound-by-sound analysis to judge the accuracy of individual sound productions. In this analysis, *there is no attempt to see a pattern in the errors* based on an underlying principle. The first approach to see a *pattern in the errors* was based on the place-voice-manner analysis. In this approach, sounds are classified into patterns based on the three phonetic features. Therefore, errors also are similarly classified. This classification resulted in somewhat *simplified patterns of errors*. The next method suggested more *complex patterns of error* classification based on distinctive features of speech sounds. Soon, however, a new approach based on *phonological theories* was proposed. *Phonological theories* proposed that phonological processes, which are patterned simplifications of speech sound productions, explain errors of articulation. These processes help classify multiple errors into groups or patterns.	The first paragraph of the first column set the stage for a historical view. But with no transition and no historical sense, the second paragraph is isolated. The first two paragraphs of the second column are related because of the common, italicized words. A theme flows from the first to the second paragraph. The third paragraph of the first column abruptly introduces the phonological process approach. The rewriting achieves smoother transition as shown by a repeated theme (italicized words in the second and the third paragraphs). The third paragraph in the first column confuses the historical sequence because of an abrupt shift to the phonological approach before mentioning the distinctive feature approach.

A.2.6b. Begin and End Most Paragraphs With Transitionary Sentences

Rough Transition	Rewrite With Smoother Transition
College students face many problems. A basic problem all college students face is lack of money. In a technological society, everyone needs a college degree to make a decent living. Unfortunately, not everyone can afford the ever-escalating cost of higher education. With limited resources, colleges are offering less financial aid to students. The rate at which the cost of higher education has escalated has outpaced that of inflation. This may be because of dwindling state support for higher education. Reduced financial aid makes it especially difficult for students with families. Balancing the needs of a family and the demand of an academic program is difficult. The difficulty is aggravated when students are faced with financial problems. Limited financial aid makes it especially difficult for students with families. *Hint:* Each paragraph contains a transitory sentence, but it is misplaced.	

Concise and Direct Writing

A.2.7a. Prefer the Shorter to the Longer Sentences

- Maintain some variety.
- Alternate longer sentences with shorter ones.

Longer Sentences	Preferred Shorter Sentences	Note
In the traditional method of articulation training, clinicians tend to use nonsense syllables in the early stages of training, along with an emphasis on ear training with a view to promote auditory discrimination of speech sounds.	In the traditional method of articulation training, clinicians tend to use nonsense syllables in the early stages of training. The training emphasis is on the ear training to promote auditory discrimination of speech sounds.	One sentence has been broken into two. These shorter sentences are easier to read and understand.
The many compounding problems of the child with a hearing loss include social isolation, academic difficulties, problems in language learning, and many others that when unchecked by a well-designed intervention plan, can lead to additional problems later in life which are then very difficult to remediate.	The many compounding problems of the child with a hearing loss include social isolation, academic difficulties, and language learning problems. Unless checked by a well-designed management plan, these problems can lead to additional difficulties later in life. Such long-standing problems are difficult to remediate.	The maze of long sentences obscures a chain of ideas or events. Some long sentences contain unnecessary words that can be cut out to shorten them.

Concise and Direct Writing

A.2.7b. Prefer the Shorter to the Longer Sentences

Longer Sentences	Rewrite in Shorter Sentences
Many clinicians, who believe that auditory training is an important part of aural rehabilitation of children with hearing loss, nonetheless do not appreciate the need for such training in case of adults with a hearing loss, though it is well established that the recognition and discrimination of speech sounds is an integral part of any program of aural rehabilitation designed for individuals of all ages.	
While the psychoanalytic theory has stated that oral and anal regression during infancy causes stuttering, the behavioral view has asserted that faulty conditioning causes it, and the neurophysiological theories have implicated either the auditory system with defective feedback loops, the laryngeal mechanism with improper neural control, or the brain with its problems in language processing in the causation of stuttering.	

A.2.8a. Prefer the Active Voice

- In the active voice, the subject of a verb performs the action (e.g., *the boy hit the ball*).
- In the passive voice, the subject of a verb is acted upon or said to receive the action (e.g., *the ball was hit by the boy*). There is nothing wrong with the passive voice; it is just that the active voice is preferable.
- Passive sentences are long and indirect.
- Active sentences make writing brief, more direct, and easier to understand.

Passive	Preferred Active
The supervisor was the person with whom I spoke.	I spoke to the supervisor.
The children were brought to the clinic by their mothers.	The mothers brought their children to the clinic.
The target responses will be modeled by the clinician.	The clinician will model the target responses.
When the target behaviors are selected, stimulus materials will be prepared.	After selecting the target behaviors, I will prepare the stimulus materials.

A.2.8b. Prefer the Active Voice

Passive	Rewrite in Preferred Active Terms
Central auditory processing problems may be assessed by various tests.	
The client's behavior problems were not controlled by the clinician.	
There are many procedures that may be used in aural rehabilitation.	
The clinician was upset by the child's uncooperative behavior.	

A.2.9a. Say What It Is, Instead of What It Is Not

- It is more direct to say what something is.
- Say it directly, even when what is said is negative.

What It Is Not	What It Is
The client often did not come to the treatment sessions at the appointed time.	The client often came late to treatment sessions.
These treatment procedures are not very effective.	These treatment procedures are ineffective.
The results of our tests do not suggest that the client does not have central auditory processing problems.	The results of our tests suggest that the client may have central auditory processing problems.
I do not believe that the client does not have a phonological disorder.	The client possibly has a phonological disorder.
I do not think that these procedures will not work with aphasia.	1. I think that these procedures might work with aphasia. 2. These procedures will work with aphasia.
The man is not honest.	The man is dishonest.
The clinician did not pay any attention to the supervisor's suggestion.	The clinician ignored the supervisor's suggestion.

A.2.9b. Say What It Is, Instead of What It Is Not

What It Is Not	What It Is
The instructor did not have much confidence in the student's explanation.	
The nativist theory does not do a great job of explaining language acquisition.	
Asking *yes/no* questions may not be an effective method of evoking continuous speech from a child.	
Some clinicians believe that phoneme auditory discrimination training may not be necessary in articulation treatment.	
Surgical procedures may not be very useful in the rehabilitation of certain types of hearing loss.	

A.2.10a. Avoid Too Many Qualifications

Too many qualifications make your writing timid, weak, and uncertain. The reader will be unsure of what you say. Let your statements be as definite as the **observations or data warrant**.

Overly Qualified and Weak	Stronger and Clearer
It is possible that some clinicians do not have a very strong belief in the validity of this theory.	1. Some clinicians doubt the validity of this theory. 2. Some clinicians reject this theory.
The data may possibly suggest that in at least some cases, the technique may have some limited use.	The data suggest that the technique may be useful in some cases.
It would be beneficial to use this assessment procedure with children, though it may or may not be just as effective with adults.	This assessment procedure may be more useful with children than with adults.
It may be possible to use the criterion of 90% correct response rate before dismissing the client.	The dismissal criterion will be 90% correct response rate.

A.2.10b. Avoid Too Many Qualifications

Overly Qualified and Weak	Stronger and Clearer
Theory may be of some value in explaining at least a small aspect of this complex phenomenon.	
I hope that with the help of this new procedure, I may be able to have some effect on the child's communication.	
I am favorably disposed to using the rate reduction procedure in the treatment of stuttering.	
I expect that I may be able to convince the parents that they may consider the possibility of holding informal treatment sessions at home.	
It is not unreasonable to expect that in all likelihood, the digital hearing aid may be of some use for this client.	

A.2.11a. Use Definite, Specific, and Concrete Language

- Avoid the overuse of generalized terms whose meanings are unclear.
- Be specific in describing symptoms of disorders, behaviors, procedures, effects, services, and so forth.

Incorrect	Correct
In all likelihood, the treatment seems to have had some positive effect on the life of the client.	Possibly, treatment helped the client speak more fluently.
Various visual and auditory stimulus input methods will be used in treatment.	Pictures, objects, action figures, and speech sound production models will be used in treatment.
I will *make sure that* the parents *support* Johnny's production of target behaviors at home.	I will ask the parents to praise Johnny for his correct production of speech sounds at home.
A variety of grammatical morphemes will be the treatment targets.	Several grammatical morphemes, including regular plurals, possessives, articles, and prepositions, will be the treatment targets.
The child was not *very cooperative* during assessment.	Often crying or whining, the child refused to name the pictures shown.
The clinician *indicated* that the client has aphasia.	The clinician said that the client has aphasia.
Children with cleft palate and their families need *numerous* services from an array of different specialists.	Children with cleft palate and their families need services from many specialists, including pediatricians, dentists, orthodontists, plastic surgeons, otologists, audiologists, speech-language pathologists, psychologists, and others.
Lack of treatment progress had some *negative effect* on the client's emotionality.	The client was disappointed because of lack of progress in treatment.
A child's improved language skills may produce many *desirable effects*.	A child's improved language skills may produce better academic performance, enriched peer interactions, and generally more efficient social communication.
I have a behavioral *issue* with the child.	The child tends to leave the chair during treatment. The child does not separate from the mother before the treatment session.

Note: In each of the correct examples, general terms such as *a variety of, various, numerous, several, many, some, positive effect, issues*, and so forth are replaced by specific terms.

A.2.11b. Use Definite, Specific, and Concrete Language

Incorrect	Write Correctly
The man with aphasia did not seem very happy during the treatment sessions. Describe behaviors that suggest unhappiness.	
Voice therapy seems to have changed the life of Mr. Shreik. Describe one or two observable changes.	
I will use any and all means of promoting response maintenance at home. Specify two or three techniques.	
The child did not want to be assessed. What did the child do?	
I will use many different procedures to assess the child's articulation. Specify two or three procedures.	
Stuttering has many kinds of effects on most aspects of life. Describe a few effects	
A child with hearing loss who has an active ear pathology needs a variety of professional services from many different specialists. Name a few services and professionals.	
The client was unfavorably disposed to continuing treatment next semester. What did the client say?	
I have issues with writing my clinical reports. Specify your problems in report writing.	

A.2.12a. Eliminate or Replace Unnecessary Phrases

Unnecessary Words	Recommendation
abilities or capabilities (unless distinguished from action)	describe actions
along the lines of	eliminate
as a matter of fact	eliminate
as far as . . . I am (we are) concerned	eliminate
as long as . . .	eliminate
at the end of the day	eliminate
at the present time	now
at this point in time	now
by means of	eliminate
call your attention to the fact that	remind you or notify you
due to the fact that	eliminate
experienced an inability	describe actions
for all intents and purposes	eliminate
hands-on experience	experience
I was unaware of the fact that	I did not know
in all honesty	eliminate
in any shape or form	eliminate
in order to	to
in spite of the fact that	eliminate
in the time frame	in about
in the area of	just name the area, topic, discipline
in the event that	if
is considered to be	eliminate
on account of the fact that	eliminate
owing to the fact that	eliminate
question as to whether	whether
the fact of the matter is	eliminate
the field of	name the discipline
there is no doubt that	no doubt, doubtless, undoubtedly
this is a subject that	this subject
to tell the truth	just say what you want to say
until such time as	until
used for the purpose of	used for (to)
with regards to, with regard to, in regard to	eliminate
with respect to	eliminate
with reference to	eliminate
when it comes to	eliminate

A.2.12b. Eliminate or Replace Unnecessary Phrases

Find at least five unnecessary phrases that people use:

1.

2.

3.

4.

5.

Write sentences containing unnecessary phrases in the first column and their revised forms in the second column.

Imprecise	Precise

A.2.12a., eliminate or replace unnecessary phrases *(continued)*

Imprecise	Precise
In the time frame of an hour, assessment may be completed.	In about an hour, assessment may be completed.
Aphasia *is considered to be* a language disorder.	Aphasia is a language disorder.
We have much controversy *in the area of* language treatment.	We have much controversy in language treatment.
Reading, writing, and speaking *abilities* were affected.	Reading, writing, and speaking were affected.
The patient *experienced an inability* to produce speech.	The patient could not produce speech.
The tongue demonstrated weakness *with regards to* lateral strength.	The tongue demonstrated lateral weakness.
A mixed probe will be *the type of* probe administered.	A mixed probe will be administered.
She *experienced great difficulty* speaking as demonstrated by slow, labored, and effortful speech.	Her speech was slow, labored, and effortful.
For *all intents and purposes*, assessment and diagnostics mean the same.	Assessment and diagnostics mean the same.
Treatment goals were not achieved *due to the fact that* the client missed several sessions.	Treatment goals were not achieved because the client missed several sessions.
On account of the fact that she was unemployed, she could not afford treatment.	Because she was unemployed, she could not afford treatment.
John won, *in spite of the fact* that he was injured.	John won, though he was injured.
We cannot offer any monetary rewards *at this point in time.*	We cannot offer any monetary rewards now.
At the present time, my case load is full.	Now my caseload is full.

A.2.12b., eliminate or replace unnecessary phrases *(continued)*

Imprecise	Write Precisely
Modeling may be considered to be an effective stimulus control procedure.	
In the area of phonological disorders, we have many assessment procedures.	
Respiration, phonation, and articulation abilities were affected.	
The patient who has a laryngectomy experiences an inability to phonate normally.	
With regard to long-term effects, loud noise is detrimental to normal hearing.	
A single-subject design will be the type of design to be used in this study.	
He experienced great difficulty in producing phonemes in sequence as demonstrated by his trial-and-error movement of the articulators.	

A.2.12a., eliminate or replace unnecessary phrases *(continued)*

Imprecise	Precise
The question as to whether all children with speech sound disorders also have phonological disorders has been debated.	Whether all children with speech sound disorders also have phonological disorders has been debated.
In the field of speech-language pathology	In speech-language pathology
He has *the ability to* lead the team.	He can lead the team.
It is good to get some *hands-on* experience in the workplace.	It is good to get some experience in the workplace.
During treatment, improvement *in terms of* the response rates was good.	During treatment, the response rates improved.
As far as the child's correct production of phonemes at home was concerned, the results were disappointing.	At home, the child did not (does not) correctly produce the phonemes.
In the event that Hector cannot complete the task, Sheila will take over.	If Hector cannot complete the task, Sheila will take over.
We will win *by means of* working harder.	We will win by working harder.
He is a man who (*she is a woman who*) knows about religion.	He (She) knows about religion.
The clinician spoke *along the lines of* normal language development.	The clinician spoke about normal language development.
With reference to mild conductive hearing loss in infancy, it may cause language delay.	Mild conductive hearing loss in infancy may cause language delay.
With respect to our earlier conversation, I will see you tomorrow.	As we talked earlier, I will see you tomorrow.
To tell you the truth, I will not be able to attend your party.	I am sorry that I cannot attend your party.
There is no doubt that he will come to the party.	He undoubtedly will come to the party.
I was unaware of the fact that she was going to bring her child.	I did not know that she was going to bring her child.
Owing to the fact that early treatment of language disorders is effective, we recommend immediate treatment for your child.	Because early treatment of language disorders is effective, we recommend immediate treatment for your child.

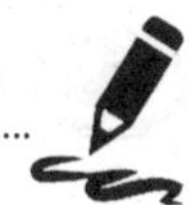

A.2.12b., eliminate or replace unnecessary phrases *(continued)*

Imprecise	Write Precisely
Morphological training was not initiated this semester due to the fact that the client did not meet the other targets.	
On account of the fact that they did not attend the IEP meetings, the parents could not be informed about the treatment targets.	
The client made excellent progress in spite of the fact that she had a severe speech sound problem.	
The fact of the matter is that many untested theories confuse the clinician.	
Our waiting list is long at this point in time.	
At the present time, all the treatment targets have been achieved.	
Until such time as the interfering behaviors are controlled, language targets cannot be trained.	
Tokens may be used for the purposes of reinforcement.	
In order to assess the client's syntactic structures, a language sample was recorded.	
The researchers have investigated the question as to whether mild conductive hearing loss in young children causes language delay.	

A.2.12a., eliminate or replace unnecessary phrases *(continued)*

Imprecise	Precise
I am very busy *until such time as* the holidays are over.	I am very busy until the holidays are over.
Our office is *used for the purposes* of distribution.	Our office is used for distribution.
In order to teach the morphological features, I will model the correct responses.	To teach the morphological features, I will model the correct responses.
I wish to call your attention to the fact that aphasia treatment is effective.	Please note that aphasia treatment is effective.
This is a subject that interests me.	This subject interests me.
When it comes to assessing children of diverse ethnocultural background, certain standardized tests may not be appropriate.	In assessing children of diverse ethnocultural background, certain standardized tests may be inappropriate.

A.2.12b., eliminate or replace unnecessary phrases *(continued)*

Imprecise	Write Precisely
The client has the ability to speak fluently.	
You can get some hands-on experience in word processing at our computer lab.	
In terms of making a complete assessment, language samples are excellent.	
As far as the client's motivation for treatment is concerned, you should make a good judgment.	
In the time frame of 20 minutes, you should administer a probe.	
In the event that the treatment sessions cannot be held twice a week, a once-a-week schedule might be tried.	
Articulation was assessed by means of the *Johnson Test of Articulation* (Johnson, 2022).	
She is a clinician who can treat persons with aphasia.	
The clinician worked along the lines of response maintenance.	
The field of audiological practice is challenging and stimulating.	
I was unaware of the fact that the client had prior therapy.	
Owing to the fact that the child has a hearing loss, there may be language delay.	
I wish to call your attention to the fact that the patient may have suffered a head injury.	
This is a subject that I am interested in doing a thesis on.	

A.2.13a. Avoid Redundant Phrases

Most redundant phrases contain two or more words that mean the same. Such phrases should be shortened, often to only one or the other word.

Redundant	Essential
future prospects	prospects
advance planning	planning
absolutely incomplete	incomplete
exactly identical	identical
repeat again	repeat *or* again
each and every	each *or* every
totally unique	unique
uniquely one of a kind	one of a kind *or* unique
reality as it is	reality
actual facts, solid facts, or true facts	facts
famous and well known	famous *or* well known
goals and objectives (when the two are not distinguished)	goals *or* objectives; *or*, distinguish the two
three different kinds, seven different varieties, or nine different types	three kinds, seven varieties, nine types
as of yet	yet
prison facilities, hospital facilities,	prison, hospital
crisis situation	crisis
problem situation	problem
prepay first	prepay *or* pay first
free gift	gift *or* free
positive growth	growth
bad weather conditions	bad weather
deteriorating client response conditions	client's deteriorating responses
positive affirmative action	affirmative action
actively involved, actively looking	involved, looking
preconditions	conditions
unexpected surprise	surprise
successfully completed	completed
successfully avoided	avoided
make an effort to try	make an effort *or* try
advice and counsel	advice *or* counsel
necessary and essential	necessary *or* essential
fair and equitable	fair *or* equitable

A.2.13b. Avoid Redundant Phrases

Find five redundant phrases used in everyday language. Suggest the essential terms.

Redundant Phrases	Essential

A.2.13a., avoid redundant phrases *(continued)*

Redundant Phrases	Essential
The *future prospects* of speech-language pathology are excellent.	The future of speech-language pathology is excellent.
NSSLHA held an *advanced planning* meeting for fundraising.	NSSLHA held a planning meeting for fundraising.
The story was *absolutely incomplete.*	The story was incomplete.
The plagiarized paper the student submitted was *exactly identical* to the original.	The plagiarized paper the student submitted was identical to the original.
Can you *repeat* that again?	Can you repeat that?
Each and every student was required to write a paper.	Each (*or* Every) student was required to write a paper.
Each client is *totally unique.*	Each client is unique.
This new test on traumatic brain injury is *uniquely one of a kind.*	This new test on traumatic brain injury is one of a kind (*or,* unique).
Outside the world of academia, *reality as it is* is different from what the professors imagine.	Outside the world of academia, reality is different from what the professors imagine.
Overgeneralization of certain words is a *true fact* of early language development.	Overgeneralization of certain words is a fact of early language development.
She is a *famous and well-known* lecturer.	She is a famous (*or* well-known) lecturer.
We should write some *goals and objectives.* *Note:* This is fine when goals are distinguished from objectives. When they are not, the phrase is redundant.	We should write some goals (*or* objectives).
We have *three different kinds of* language tests.	We have three kinds of language tests.
It is not done *as of yet.*	It is not done yet.
We will visit the *prison facilities.*	We will visit the prison.
We have a *crisis situation* on hand.	We have a crisis on hand.
Deteriorating client *response conditions* were distressing.	Deteriorating client responses were distressing.
There were some *pre*conditions for negotiation.	There were some conditions for negotiation.

A.2.13b., avoid redundant phrases *(continued)*

Redundant Phrases	Essential
The future prospects of maintenance of fluency are excellent.	
The officers held an advanced planning meeting.	
The treatment report was absolutely incomplete.	
The two stimuli used on treatment and probe trials were exactly identical.	
The clinician will repeat modeling again.	
Each and every client's family members should be trained in response maintenance.	
For each client, we do not need totally unique treatment procedures.	
I found uniquely one-of-a-kind software for surfing the internet.	
Reality as it is may be more disappointing than we imagine it to be.	
An actual fact of clinical practice is some degree of apprehension.	
He is a famous and well-known author.	
My treatment goals and objectives were not clear.	

A.2.13a., avoid redundant phrases *(continued)*

Redundant Phrases	Essential
She is *actively looking* for a job.	She is looking for a job.
We had an *unexpected surprise* in therapy session.	We had a surprise in therapy session.
She *successfully completed* our graduate program.	She completed our graduate program.
I will make an *effort to try* to train parents in response maintenance.	I will try to train parents in response maintenance.
A *necessary and essential* element of treatment is positive reinforcement.	A necessary (*or* essential) element of treatment is positive reinforcement.
The grading was *fair and equitable.*	The grading was fair (*or* equitable).

A.2.13b., avoid redundant phrases *(continued)*

Redundant Phrases	Essential
We have three different types of assignments in the class.	
We offer 11 different varieties of language treatment.	
The treatment program is not complete as of yet.	
We will visit the prison facilities.	
The problem situation is getting worse.	
The bad weather conditions were getting worse.	
I did not accept their preconditions for employment.	
My client is actively involved in the treatment process.	
The child's sudden temper tantrum was an unexpected surprise to me.	
The client successfully completed all steps in the treatment.	
She made an effort to try to keep the appointment.	
Paperwork is a necessary and essential element of professional practice.	
The pay raise offered to us was fair and equitable.	

A.2.14a. Avoid Wordiness

Wordiness is the use of unnecessary words resulting in vague, timid, and unnecessarily long sentences.

Wordy	Precise	Note
It seems to me that it certainly is very important to consider many factors in selecting treatment procedures.	I should consider many factors in selecting treatment procedures.	It is even better to specify a few factors that need to be considered.
It became evident from my conversation with the parents of the child that they had a very difficult time to do what they were told to do because of their busy lifestyle.	The parents of the child told me that they did not have time to conduct treatment sessions at home.	Fewer words specify the problem.
Although the client was certainly not negatively disposed to continuing the treatment for a reasonable amount of time, she finally decided to discontinue it.	The client discontinued the treatment, though she said she wanted to continue it.	The overused word *certainly* often suggests no certainty.
There were several crucial factors that led me to select these assessment procedures.	These assessment procedures were selected because of their known reliability, validity, and simplicity.	Often, the word *crucial* is an overstatement.
A variety of procedures will be used.	Many procedures will be used.	Procedures may be specified in subsequent sentences.
A number of clients were treated.	Several clients were treated.	It is assumed that the exact number is unimportant.
Certain limitations of standardized tests make it imperative to carefully reconsider the whole issue of reliability and validity of assessment procedures.	Because of the limitations of standardized tests, we should reconsider the reliability and validity of assessment procedures.	Limitations will have been specified.
It is not in the least inappropriate to offer the suggestion that cochlear implant may be a reasonably attractive method of aural rehabilitation that should not be rejected out of hand.	The option of cochlear implant should be considered.	The more precise statement says it positively as well.

A.2.14b. Avoid Wordiness

Wordy	Rewrite Precisely
In my judgment, it is reasonable to conclude that there are different types of aphasia though many symptoms are common to the different types.	
I personally think that it is not totally inappropriate to suggest that children with multiple misarticulations have a phonological disorder.	
I used two tests that were known to have a reasonable degree of reliability.	
It certainly seems to me that we need more treatment efficacy research.	
A variety of investigators have found it appropriate to suggest that both genetic and environmental factors play a causative role in stuttering.	
It is not unreasonable to suggest that we carefully consider all minimally attractive alternatives available to us at this important juncture.	
It is certainly apparent to most competent clinicians that it is reasonably worthwhile to offer voice therapy to certain clients who may wish to consider it as an attractive alternative to surgical procedures.	
If one were to infer from these assessment data that the client has Broca's aphasia, the inference would certainly not seem totally inappropriate.	

A.2.15a. Avoid Jargon

- *Jargon* is a technical or specialized term, often unavoidable in scientific, professional, and technical writing.
- Do not overuse jargon.
- When necessary, describe what jargon means in everyday language.
- When you write to or speak to people without technical knowledge, describe everything in nontechnical terms; if necessary, introduce the technical terms accompanied by nontechnical descriptions.
- When writing to technical audiences, retain the technical terms but define them.

<table>
<tr><th>Jargon</th><th>Plain</th><th>Note</th></tr>
<tr><td>The child's linguistic competence is limited.</td><td>The child's language is limited.</td><td rowspan="4">In some cases, there may not be a need to introduce the technical terms at all.</td></tr>
<tr><td>Use an FR2 schedule to reinforce correct responses at home.</td><td>Reinforce every other correct response at home.</td></tr>
<tr><td>In using your hearing aid, learn to control the intensity of the signal.</td><td>In using your hearing aid, learn to control the volume.</td></tr>
<tr><td>The child's MLU is limited.</td><td>The child speaks in short phrases or sentences.</td></tr>
<tr><td>The woman has anomia.</td><td>The woman has naming difficulties. It is called anomia.</td><td rowspan="3">Examples in which technical terms also are introduced.</td></tr>
<tr><td>A patient with a stroke may have dysphagia.</td><td>A patient with a stroke may have difficulty swallowing. It is called dysphagia.</td></tr>
<tr><td>The child has a phonological disorder.</td><td>The child has difficulty producing certain speech sounds correctly. This difficulty is known as a phonological disorder.</td></tr>
<tr><td>Jenny should be praised for her correct use of morphological features.</td><td>Jenny should be praised for her correct use of plural or past tense inflections.</td><td>The clinician should then go on to give examples.</td></tr>
</table>

A.2.15b. Avoid Jargon

Jargon	Write in Plain Language
The boy has a severe problem in correctly positioning his articulators. *Hint:* Difficulty producing speech sounds.	
The child has telegraphic speech. *Hint:* Omits certain grammatical features.	Introduce the technical term.
The woman has aphonia.	Introduce the technical term.
The child has a final consonant deletion process.	Introduce the technical term.
The man has Wernicke's aphasia. *Hint:* Fluent speech but poor understanding of spoken language.	Introduce the technical term.
The woman has apraxia of speech. *Hint:* Difficulty producing speech sounds in proper sequence.	Introduce the technical term.
The child has a specific language impairment. *Hint:* Only a language problem, no other problems.	

A.2.16a. Avoid Euphemism

- Euphemistic expressions disguise negative meanings.
- Such expressions falsely suggest neutral or positive meanings.
- Euphemistic writing can be dishonest.

Euphemistic	Direct
Because of poor progress, the family will be *counseled out* of our services.	1. Because of poor progress, the family will be dismissed from our services. 2. Because of poor progress, we recommended to the family that our services be discontinued.
The client is *communicatively challenged.*	1. The client has a communication disorder. 2. The client stutters.
The child comes from an *economically deprived* background.	The child comes from a poor family.
The clinic reported *negative profits* for the third quarter.	1. The clinic reported a loss of revenue for the third quarter. 2. The clinic lost money during the third quarter.
The child is *developmentally other-abled.*	1. The child has intellectual disabilities. 2. The child has a developmental disability. *Note:* The term *intellectual disabilities* is preferred.
He is a *residentially challenged* person.	He is a homeless person.
The treatment had *negative outcomes.*	1. The treatment was ineffective. 2. The treatment was harmful to the clients.
The army reported *collateral damage* from the bombings.	1. The army reported civilian casualties resulting from the bombings. 2. The bombs killed civilians and destroyed their homes.
The government announced new *revenue enhancement measures.*	The government increased taxes.
Children with *special needs* require special services.	1. Children with disabilities need special services. 2. Gifted children need special services.
The parents were less than cooperative in maintaining their child's fluency at home.	The parents did little or no work at home to maintain their child's fluency.

A.2.16b. Avoid Euphemism

Euphemistic	Write More Directly
The student was counseled out of the major.	
The child comes from an underprivileged family.	
The man is physically challenged.	
Today, the garbologist did not collect the trash.	
I bought a previously owned car.	
After evaluating your performance in the comprehensive examination, we have decided to give you another wonderful opportunity to demonstrate your outstanding knowledge.	
The surgical treatment had a negative outcome for the patient.	
The arbor technician pruned the fruit trees.	
I made negative profits from my home-based business.	
I found the parents less than helpful in helping the child complete home assignments.	

A.2.17a. Keep Related Words Together

- Do not split related words by introducing intervening words.
- Keep the conceptually related words adjacent to each other.

Incorrect	Correct	Note
He ate seven hot dogs for lunch last Friday, and three more for dinner.	Last Friday, he ate seven hot dogs for lunch and three more for dinner.	Makes it clear that he ate the hot dogs for lunch and dinner on the same day.
An unruly behavior of a child, if you do not control it, will prevent rapid progress in treatment.	Unless controlled, a child's unruly behavior will prevent rapid progress in treatment.	What prevents rapid progress?
Treatment of cluttering, because of limited research, is not well established.	Because of limited research, treatment of cluttering is not well established.	What is not well established?
Some clinicians, though they are keenly interested in it, are not well trained in the assessment of dysphagia.	Although they are keenly interested in dysphagia, some clinicians are not well trained in its assessment.	In what are the clinicians not well trained?
The supervisor asked clinicians to write a treatment plan for each client at the meeting on Wednesday.	At the meeting on Wednesday, the supervisor asked clinicians to write a treatment plan for each client.	Clinicians did not write a treatment plan at the meeting itself.
This is an assessment report on Mr. Davis, referred to us by Dr. Benson, seen last week in our facility.	This is an assessment report on Mr. Davis, seen last week in our facility. He was referred to us by Dr. Benson.	Dr. Benson was not seen last week!
Women who are pregnant, but unaware of its bad effects, may continue to drink alcohol.	Women who are pregnant, but unaware of the bad effects of alcohol on the fetus, may continue to drink.	Bad effects of drinking or pregnancy?
The human fertility clinic extracted multiple ova from women, then froze them.	The human fertility clinic extracted multiple ova from women. The clinic then froze the ova.	Ova, not women, were frozen!

Note: See also A.1.16a and A.2.21a about the correct use of modifiers.

A.2.17b. Keep Related Words Together

Incorrect	Write Correctly
Maintenance of target behaviors, if not carefully programmed, will not be achieved.	
In assessing phonological disorders, though many procedures may be appropriate, conversational speech is the most productive.	
Meeting the IEP goals within 3 months, even if I work hard and the child is regular for sessions, will be difficult.	
The selected target behaviors may be taught, assuming that the client will be regular for treatment sessions, in about 10 sessions.	
The final target of treatment, it has been suggested, is maintenance.	
The treatment procedure will include generalized reinforcers, to make it more effective.	
Clinicians who are inexperienced, but do not know how hazardous it is, may cause serious problems by using wrong methods of dysphagia treatment.	
I wrote this treatment plan for Mrs. Jones, after careful consideration of her strengths and weaknesses.	

Parallelism

A.2.18a. Write in Parallel Terms

- Parallelism is the expression of a series of ideas in the same grammatical form.
- Parallelism is broken when some ideas in a series are expressed in one form and the others in the same series are expressed in different forms.

Incorrect	Correct	Note
Children with language disorders tend to be deficient in their use of grammatical morphemes, syntactic structures, and *they also may have a limited vocabulary.*	Children with language disorders tend to be deficient in their use of grammatical morphemes, syntactic structures, and complex words.	The incorrect versions have a *nonparallel final clause.* The correct versions restore parallelism to the final clause.
The child with hearing loss has difficulty speaking, reading, and *self-confidence.*	The child with hearing loss has difficulty speaking, reading, and maintaining self-confidence.	
Disadvantages of primary reinforcers include satiation, dietary restriction, and *they also are difficult to administer to groups.*	Disadvantages of primary reinforcers include satiation, dietary restriction, and problematic group administration.	
Parental reinforcement of target behaviors helps maintenance by *not* allowing extinction, strengthening the behaviors, and increasing their use in natural environments.	Parental reinforcement of target behaviors helps maintenance by *not* allowing extinction, by strengthening the behaviors, and by increasing their use in natural environments.	The incorrect version is nonparallel because the word *not* applies only to the first in the series. In the correct version, the repetition of *by* restores parallelism.
The target behaviors, the stimuli, and reinforcers, should all be specified.	The target behaviors, the stimuli, and the reinforcers should all be specified.	An article is either repeated before all parallel terms, or is used only before the first term. (The target behaviors, stimuli, and reinforcers . . .)

Parallelism

A.2.18b. Write in Parallel Terms

Incorrect	Write Correctly
Many persons who stutter have been frustrated in the past because the therapists lacked adequate training, supervised experience, and the therapists' scientific knowledge of stuttering has been limited.	
Persons with communicative problems have difficulty talking, reading, and self-confidence.	
Some of the side effects of saying "no" to a client include aggression, reticence, and the client may also feel resentment toward the clinician.	
To promote response maintenance, I will select stimuli from the client's home, train self-monitoring skills, teach target behavior charting, and parent training will also be included.	
Persons with aphasia may be treated with auditory stimulation and verbal expression also may be taught.	
The theory may be criticized for three reasons: first, it is illogical; second, it is nonempirical; third, it is also difficult to apply.	
The client may receive treatment in fall, spring, or in summer terms. *Hint:* The preposition is either repeated before all terms or used before the first term only.	

A.2.19a. Maintain Parallelism in Numbered or Bulleted Lists

Incorrect	Correct	Note
Today's treatment objectives will include • training the /s/ in the word final positions • working on naming skills • oral-motor exercises.	Today's treatment objectives include • training the /s/ in the word final positions • working on naming skills • providing oral-motor exercises	Incorrect mixing of verb phrases with noun phrases in a list is corrected; this is a common mistake in numbered or bulleted lists.
Assessment will include the following steps: 1. hearing screening 2. orofacial examination 3. language sampling 4. any special tests that need to be administered should also be considered	Assessment will include the following steps: 1. hearing screening 2. orofacial examination 3. language sampling 4. special test administration (if any)	
In treating children, specialists recommend that you • speak in simple terms • choose client-specific stimuli • select reinforcers • parent training also should be considered	In treating children, specialists recommend that you • speak in simple terms • choose client-specific stimuli • select reinforcers • train parents	
Characteristics of motherese include • slower rate of speech • greater pitch variations • simpler words • higher speech fluency • articulation may be clear	Characteristics of motherese include • slower rate of speech • greater pitch variations • simpler words • higher speech fluency • clearer articulation	

A.2.19b. Maintain Parallelism in Numbered or Bulleted Lists

Incorrect	Write Correctly
Children with language disorders show the following four major problems: 1. poor listening skills 2. limited understanding of word meanings 3. limited verbal expressions 4. narrative skills also may be impaired	
Research on speech sound acquisition has shown that • vowels are acquired before consonants • stops are mastered earlier than fricatives • nasals are mastered before affricates • consonant clusters may take the longest to be acquired	
To promote response maintenance, I will • select stimuli from the client's home • train self-monitoring skills • teach target behavior charting • parent training will be included	
The problems associated with cleft palate in children include • feeding problems • middle ear infections • dental problems • parents may have negative emotional reactions	

Misplaced or Dangling Modifiers

A.2.20a. Avoid Dangling Modifiers

- Dangling modifiers often do not seem to modify anything in a sentence.
- A phrase that is better placed at the beginning of a sentence may be left dangling at the end.

Incorrect	Correct	Note
The clinician selected children for treatment, *taking into consideration the eligibility criteria.*	*Taking into consideration the eligibility criteria,* the clinician selected children for treatment.	In most cases, dangling phrases can be fixed by moving them to an earlier position in the sentence.
Many undesirable effects of amplification have been eliminated, *with the use of digital hearing aids.*	1. *With the use of digital hearing aids, audiologists* have eliminated many undesirable effects of amplification. 2. Audiologists have shown that *digital hearing aids* eliminate many undesirable effects of amplification.	Correct versions are in active voice; hence, they are more direct.
I will teach the client self-monitoring skills, *to promote maintenance.*	*To promote maintenance,* I will teach the client self-monitoring skills.	
Children's language problems should not be ignored, *because they can lead to academic failure.*	*Because they can lead to academic failure,* we should not ignore children's language problems.	Active voice.

Misplaced or Dangling Modifiers

A.2.20b. Avoid Dangling Modifiers

Incorrect	Write Correctly
I selected assessment procedures, giving much thought to reliability and validity.	
The problems of response maintenance may be handled, using parent training programs.	
Hearing will be tested, with an appropriately calibrated audiometer. *Hint:* Specify who will test the hearing.	
Ten children will be selected for the study, all with cochlear implants. *Hint:* Specify who will select the children.	
I will teach the child several phonemes this semester, to eliminate their speech sound disorder.	
Alzheimer's disease profoundly affects everyone involved, because it changes everything for the affected person and the family.	

A.2.21a. Avoid Misplaced Modifiers

- Misplaced modifiers seem to modify the wrong word in a sentence.
- Move the modifier closer to the word it correctly modifies.

<table>
<tr><th>Incorrect</th><th>Correct</th><th>Note</th></tr>
<tr><td>Based on the hypothesis, Erickson developed his theory.</td><td>The theory that Erickson developed was based on this hypothesis.</td><td>Erickson was not based on the hypothesis.</td></tr>
<tr><td>In the study, these assumptions were only tested partially in the study.</td><td>In the study, these assumptions were tested only partially.</td><td rowspan="2">The misplaced word only is moved closer to the word it modifies.</td></tr>
<tr><td>The experimental group scored 10, but the control group only scored 5.</td><td>The experimental group scored 10, but the control group scored only 5.</td></tr>
</table>

A.2.21b. Avoid Misplaced Modifiers

Incorrect	Correct
Based on this evidence, I developed a treatment.	
Only the evidence partially supported the theory.	
The adults gained 10 points whereas the children only gained 4 points.	

Shifts Within and Between Sentences

A.2.22a. Avoid Shifts Within and Between Sentences

- Unless justified, do not shift tense, voice, and mood within or between sentences.
- Do not shift number within or between sentences.

Incorrect	Correct	Note
The clinician *was* well trained. She *knows* how to treat a variety of disorders. Nevertheless, she *had* difficulty treating this client.	The clinician *was* well trained. She *knew* how to treat a variety of disorders. Nevertheless, she *had* difficulty treating this client.	A shift in tense (in a group of sentences or in a single sentence) is corrected by maintaining the same past or present tense.
The story *talks* about a man and woman who *fell* in love.	The story *talks* about a man and woman who *fall* in love.	
Van Riper first *developed* an eclectic theory, and later a more integrative theory was also *proposed.*	Van Riper first *developed* an eclectic theory and later *proposed* a more integrative theory.	A shift from active to passive voice is corrected by maintaining the active voice.
When *one* is reviewing the literature, *you* find that few studies exist.	When *one* is reviewing the literature, *one* finds that few studies exist.	A shift from second to third person is corrected by maintaining the same pronoun form.
If a *student* studies hard, *you* will impress teachers.	1. If a *student* studies hard, *he* or *she* will impress teachers.	A third to second person shift is corrected.
	2. If a *student* studies hard, *they* will impress teachers.	Acceptable plural *they* to refer back to a singular noun.
	3. A student who studies hard will impress teachers.	This may be the most preferred.
All *hospitals* have *a* physician.	All hospitals have physicians.	A shift from plural to singular is corrected by maintaining the plural.
It is important that an author *buy* a computer and *uses* it regularly.	It is important that an author *buy* a computer and *use* it regularly.	A shift in mood is corrected by maintaining the same imperative mood.

Shifts Within and Between Sentences

A.2.22b. Avoid Shifts Within and Between Sentences

Incorrect	Write Correctly
The client was highly motivated for treatment. Therefore, the progress is good.	
I will first train grammatical morphemes. Later, syntactic features also will be trained.	
When one considers treatment options, you find many alternatives.	
A review shows that this type of experiment has not been conducted. The review also has shown that it is difficult to control all the variables.	
The data suggested that the method was effective. The response rate indicates that maintenance also is enhanced.	
All public schools have a speech-language pathologist.	
If a clinician is exceptional, you are likely to get promoted.	
It is important that a clinician buy recent books and studied them carefully.	
The supervisor observed the client, and then talks to the parent.	

Quotations

A.2.23a. Make Quotations Count

- Select only effective and memorable phrases to quote.
- Do not quote descriptive and ordinary statements.

<table>
<tr><th>Descriptive and Ordinary</th><th>Rewritten Without Quotations</th><th>Note</th></tr>
<tr><td>Not all communication disorders are related to environmental variables. Research has shown that “many genetic syndromes are associated with communication disorders” (Brightly, 2022, p. 25).</td><td>Not all communication disorders are related to environmental variables. Research has shown that several genetic syndromes may be related to communication disorders (Brightly, 2022).</td><td rowspan="5">Rephrase the quotations that do not say anything worth quoting.

Do not just remove the quote marks, rephrase it in your own terms.

Give reference to specific source of information.

Although common-knowledge or general statements do not need a reference, it may be prudent to give one in scientific writing.

Note that even common-knowledge or general statements found in a source should be rephrased to avoid plagiaristic writing.</td></tr>
<tr><td>According to Qotme, “aphasia is a common language disorder found in the older population” (2012, p. 9).</td><td>Among older people, aphasia is a common language disorder (Qotme, 2012).</td></tr>
<tr><td>Quotman stated that “many neurological conditions can be associated with speech and language disorders” (2020, p. 589).</td><td>Speech and language disorders may be correlated with many neurological diseases or problems (Quotman, 2020).</td></tr>
<tr><td>Communication disorders have a significant effect on the “social, occupational, and personal life of an individual” (Wisdon, 2019, p. 28).</td><td>Communication disorders negatively affect an individual’s personal, occupational, and social life (Wisdon, 2019).</td></tr>
<tr><td>According to Surveyor, “roughly 10% of the population may have a communication disorder” (2016, p. 18).</td><td>It is believed that one or more communicative disorders may be found in 10% of the population (Surveyor, 2016).</td></tr>
</table>

Quotations

A.2.23b. Make Quotations Count

In rewriting the passages, do not just remove the quotation marks from the statements; rewrite them in your words. If you simply remove the quotation marks, the writing will be plagiaristic.

Descriptive and Ordinary	Rewrite Without Quotations
According to Linguistron, "many school-age children have language disorders that go undetected" (2017, p. 50).	
Many researchers have studied "the relation between mild conductive hearing loss and language development" (Otiss, 2015, p. 19).	
During hearing testing, "the clinician should mask the better ear" (Noisley, 2015, p. 567).	
According to Effecton, "some treatment procedures are effective while others are not" (2016, p. 20).	
Brimm has stated that "language acquisition is a complex process" (2005, p. 23).	
"Speech sound disorders are common among school-age children" (Soundman, 2012, p. 20).	

A.2.24a. Do Not Overuse Quotations

- Do not use quotations to reduce the amount of your writing.
- Unless a quote is memorable, paraphrase it and give credit.
- Limit the number of quotations to no more than just a few in any paper you write.
- Minimize the use of long (block) quotations.

Overuse	Judicious Use	Note
The study of language has shown "many rapid changes over the years" (Thomas, 2010, p. 90). In the 1940s, "descriptive linguistics dominated the study of language" (TeNiel, 2005, p. 13). According to Thomas (2010), the focus shifted to "transformational generative grammar in the late 1950s and early 1960s" (p. 118). Then again in the 1970s, the focus was shifted to "the essence of language: meaning" (Revolutionary, 2015, p. 50). Soon, however, this approach was abandoned in favor of a "new pragmatic approach" (Bomber, 2016, p. 120).	During the past few decades, the study of language has changed many times. In the 1940s, descriptive linguistics was the main approach. Dissatisfied with a purely descriptive study, Chomsky (1957) and others in the late 1950s proposed a new transformational generative grammar approach. In the 1970s, those who disagreed with the purely theoretical grammar approach proposed a new semantic view that focused on "the essence of language: meaning" (Revolutionary, 2015, p. 50). Soon, this, too, was replaced by the newer pragmatic approach (Bomber, 2016).	Overuse of quotations tends to include unremarkable statements as well. Writing littered with ineffective quotes is difficult to read.
Some question whether "apraxia of speech exists in children at all" (Smoothly, 2014, p. 27). In adults, apraxia is "associated with observable signs of neurological disease or trauma" (Brain, 2016, p. 25). Head (1929) has stated that when there is no evidence of neurological involvement, "apraxia of speech in children is a doubtful diagnostic classification" (p. 19).	Some question the existence of apraxia of speech in children. In adults who have apraxia of speech, symptoms of neurological diseases or trauma are documented. Therefore, in the absence of neurological involvement, diagnosis of apraxia in children is questionable (Brain, 2016; Head, 1929; Smoothly, 2014).	

A.2.24b. Do Not Overuse Quotations

In rewriting the passages, do not just eliminate the quotation marks. Rephrase the information.

Overuse	Rewrite With Fewer Quotations
Inappropriate behavior causes several forms of voice disorders. According to Scream, "how you use your voice will determine whether you will have a healthy voice or not" (2008, p. 90). Loud (2013) also stated that "certain occupations pose high risk for voice disorders" (p. 13). Shout said a prudent person avoids "noisy places" (2009, p. 118).	
Either the right or the left ear may be tested first because "the selection is purely arbitrary" (Horton, 2014, p. 32). Research has not shown that it is "better to test one or the other ear first" (McClauey, 2015, p. 67). Most audiologists "begin testing at 1000 Hz, though the order in which the frequencies are tested may not be important" (Soundson, 2016, p. 45). Some audiologists "do not test at 125 Hz at all, while others do" (Southern, 2007, p. 22).	

A.2.25a. Do Not Include Islands of Quotations

- Do not let quotations stand alone in your writing.
- Blend quotations smoothly into your expressions.
- Write phrases that lead to the quotation.
- On occasion, write your own words after the quotation.

Incorrect	Correct	Note
Autism spectrum is a serious childhood disorder. It starts in early childhood. "Children who are autistic do not live in the world of their families, but in their own world of distorted fantasy" (Scitzmoore, 2015, p. 10). The disorder affects thought and language. "Children who are autistic are unable to form emotional bonds with their loved ones" (Sentiment, 2013, p. 15). This can cause serious interpersonal problems.	Autism spectrum is a serious childhood disorder. It starts in early childhood. Children with autism spectrum are not in touch with their surroundings as they seem to live "in their own world of distorted fantasy" Scitzmoore, 2015, p. 10). The disorder affects thought, language, and emotional experience. According to Sentiment (2013), the children who are autistic are "unable to form emotional bonds with their loved ones" (p. 15), resulting in serious interpersonal problems.	You quote fewer words when you integrate quotations with your writing. In the correct version, no quotation stands alone. Phrases such as *according to*, *as stated by*, *as written by*, and *the author stated that* lead the reader to the quotation and help blend a quotation with the main writing.

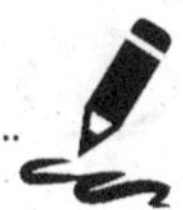

A.2.25b. Do Not Include Islands of Quotations

Incorrect	Write Correctly
Multiple misarticulations suggest a need for a phonological pattern analysis. "A pattern analysis helps the clinician see order in what might appear to be a collection of random errors" (Godsen, 2015, p. 45). Several methods of phonological analysis are available. "The clinician should select the one that is simple to use and comprehensive in its analysis" (Nixon, 2017, p. 10).	

A.2.26a. Do Not Begin a Sentence With a Quotation

- Begin sentences with your words.
- Insert quotations within or at the end of your sentence.

Incorrect	Correct
"Cleft palate speech is most readily recognized" (Milton, 2015, p. 20) because of its unique characteristics.	Because of its unique characteristics, "cleft palate speech is most readily recognized" (Milton, 2015, p. 20).
"In recent years, computerized audiometers have been developed to automatically control all aspects of pure tone air- and bone-conduction testing" (Robotson, 2005, p. 98); however, this does not mean that we "do not need audiologists who have a good clinical sense" (Robotson, 2005, p. 99).	In recent years, the administration of hearing tests has been computerized. However, as pointed out by Robotson (2005), we still need audiologists "who have a good clinical sense" (p. 99).

A.2.26b. Do Not Begin a Sentence With a Quotation

Incorrect	Write Correctly
“Audiometers alone, no matter how advanced, will not diagnose hearing loss” (Torkin, 2016, p. 32). It is the clinician’s expert interpretation of results that leads to a clinical diagnosis. “No mechanical device is a substitute for good clinical sense” (Barkin, 2017, p. 551).	
“Specific language impairment often is not associated with an identifiable cause” (Barney, 2014, p. 40). The child may be normal in every respect except for delayed language. “It is hypothesized that specific language delay may have a genetic basis” (Tomokin, 2013, p. 22).	

A.2.27a. Use Quotation and Punctuation Marks Correctly

- Enclose all direct quotations within two double quotations marks (“and”).
- Use single quotation marks (‘and’) to enclose a quotation within a quotation.
- In most cases, place the punctuation mark *within* the quotation mark; take note of an exception in the last example.
- Double-check for missing quotation marks at the beginning or the ending of quotations.

<table>
<tr><th>Incorrect</th><th>Correct</th><th>Note</th></tr>
<tr><td>The clinician said, “Good job”.</td><td>The clinician said, “Good job.”</td><td rowspan="4">The first two incorrect versions have the punctuation marks outside the quotation marks.
The last two have missing quotation marks.
Exception to the punctuation rule: When a reference citation follows a quotation, the period is placed after the closing parenthesis.</td></tr>
<tr><td>I will say “wrong”, and then mark the incorrect response on the sheet.</td><td>I will say “wrong,” and then mark the incorrect response on the sheet.</td></tr>
<tr><td>He said that he was “sorry for what happened.</td><td>He said that he was “sorry for what happened.”</td></tr>
<tr><td>According to Soundson, hearing loss costs billions of dollars to the nation’s health care system.” (2010, p. 9).</td><td>According to Soundson, “hearing loss costs billions of dollars to the nation’s health care system” (2010, p. 9).</td></tr>
</table>

A.2.27b. Use Quotation and Punctuation Marks Correctly

Incorrect	Write Correctly
Mrs. Aktsungfoong added that her husband is "stubborn" and "difficult to manage".	
The parents said that their son is "delighted", "very pleased", and "impressed" with the services.	
One expert stated that "remediating pragmatic language disorders is the most important treatment target".	

A.2.28a. Do Not Misuse Quotation Marks

Do not enclose book and journal titles, technical terms, terms of special emphasis, and linguistic examples within quotation marks; use italics as shown.

Incorrect	Correct	Note
"Aphasia: A clinical approach."	*Aphasia: A clinical approach.*	A book title or a journal name is italicized.
"American Journal of Audiology"	*American Journal of Audiology*	
"Dysphonia" means disordered voice.	*Dysphonia* means disordered voice. **Dysphonia** means disordered voice.	When it is defined, a technical term may be in italics or boldface.
You may not always substitute the conjunction "and" for the ampersand "&."	You may not always substitute the conjunction *and* for the ampersand &.	Linguistic examples are italicized (not bolded).

Exception: The titles of articles and research papers are neither enclosed within quotation marks nor italicized. However, titles of theses and dissertations (published or unpublished) are italicized.

A.2.28b. Do Not Misuse Quotation Marks

Incorrect	Write Correctly
"Introduction to Audiology" by Matson	
"Journal of Speech, Language, and Hearing Research"	
"Congenital disorder" is a disorder noticed at the time of birth or soon thereafter.	
The child does not produce the possessive "s" and the present progressive "ing."	

A.2.29a. Give References for All Direct Quotations

In scientific writing, all direct quotations should include the following:

- the last name of the author or authors
- the year of publication
- the number of the page or pages on which the quotation is found

Incorrect	Correct	Note
According to Confusius, "a terrible confusion between who you are and what you want to be" causes stuttering.	According to Confusius (2002), "a terrible confusion between who you are and what you want to be" (p. 37) causes stuttering.	The incorrect version includes neither the year of publication nor the page number.
Mixtupton recommended that "children with phonological disorders should be separated from those with a mere articulation disorder" (2015).	Mixtupton (2015) recommended that "children with phonological disorders should be separated from those with a mere articulation disorder" (p. 23).	The incorrect version includes the year of publication but omits the page number.
It has been stated that "chronic and excessively loud speech is detrimental to healthy voice."	It has been stated that "chronic and excessively loud speech is detrimental to healthy voice" (Louden, 2012, p. 10).	The worst of the three, this incorrect version omits the author's name, year of publication, and the page number.
Although persons who stutter may show some excessive anxiety, it is "often associated with speech, and, therefore, there is no evidence for a "trait anxiety" in most stutterers" (Angst, 2011, p. 67).	Although persons who stutter may show some excessive anxiety, it is "often associated with speech, and, therefore, there is no evidence for a 'trait anxiety' in most stutterers" (Angst, 2011, p. 67).	A phrase with double quotation marks within a quotation is enclosed within single quotation marks.
Although found in all societies, "the incidence of cleft palate varies across different racial groups, suggesting the importance of genetic factors in its etiology" (Geneson, 2013, p. 10–11).	Although found in all societies, "the incidence of cleft palate varies across different racial groups, suggesting the importance of genetic factors in its etiology" (Geneson, 2013, pp. 10–11).	The correct version shows the page on which the quotation begins and the page on which it ends. Use p. for one page and pp. for two or more pages, both in lowercase.

Note: There are different methods of placing the name, the year, and the page number. The period is placed only after the parenthetical closure, not before or after the quotation marks.

A.2.29b. Give References for All Direct Quotations

Invent the information that is needed to correct the statements.

Incorrect	Write Correctly
According to Loveson, many factors cause language delay, "but none can be directly traced to lack of parental love for the child."	
Boontenthorpe has written that "adults who have strokes and aphasia show remarkable spontaneous recovery within 3 to 6 months of onset" (2014).	
It has been stated that "a single, loud scream can damage the vocal folds."	
A neglected cause of hearing loss is "the types of food we eat; it is possible that "pesticide- laced" grains and fruits are a source of cochlear damage in some cases" (Peston, 2011, p. 67). *Hint:* A quote within a quote.	
Recent developments in cochlear implants have "made it possible for many deaf children to begin their aural rehabilitation early in life" (Coplant, 2015, p. 15–16). *Hint:* Page range.	

A.2.30a. Reproduce Quotations Exactly

- Make quotations identical to the original in words, spelling, and punctuation.
- Reproduce errors as they are in the original with the insertion of the word [*sic*], italicized, and placed within brackets.

A Quotation With an Error in It	Note
Numbasa's description of language as a mental phenomenon "that can be studied only by some powerfil [*sic*] intuitive procedures" was especially appealing to clinicians who had based their treatment procedures on intuition.	In the quotation, the italicized word [*sic*] suggests that in the original, the word *powerful* is misspelled.

A.2.31a. Integrate Quotations of Fewer Than 40 Words With the Text

Incorrect (Unintegrated)	Correct	Note
Mentalis defined language as: "A cognitive ability to synthesize and symbolize mental experience and to represent this experience in patterns of sounds, words, and sentences following linguistic rules that are innately given" (2014, p. 95). Cognitive psychologists and linguists who think that speaking a language is not action, but a mental process widely cite Mentalis's definition.	Mentalis (2014) defined language as "a cognitive ability to synthesize and symbolize mental experience and to represent this experience in patterns of sounds, words, and sentences following linguistic rules that are innately given" (p. 95). Cognitive psychologists and linguists who think that speaking a language is not action but a mental process widely cite Mentalis's definition.	Only quotations of 40 words or more are set off from the rest of the text as *block* quotations. See A.2.32.

A.2.30b. Reproduce Quotations Exactly

Quotation With an Error in it	Quote it Appropriately
Softhead (2015) said that "language is not to be confused with what people say, because language is a metal tool of imagination" (p. 40). *Hint: metal* or *mental*?	

A.2.31b. Integrate Quotations of Fewer Than 40 Words With the Text

Incorrectly Arranged Quotation	Integrate the Quote With Text
Nullbrain (2015) stated that: Every child who learns to speak his or her language is a scientist who tests alternative hypotheses about the nature of language. The utterances the child hears are the data for hypothesis testing. (p. 23) Critics have contended that such statements betray a theoretical fantasy. *Hint:* A 33-word quotation	*Hint:* Write a single paragraph containing the quotation.

A.2.32a. Arrange Quotations as a *Block* When They Have 40 Words or More

- A quotation set apart from the text is a *block quotation.*
- Set quotations of 40 words or more as block quotations.
- Indent the entire quotation by five spaces from the left margin, as for a new paragraph.
- Indent the first line of the second (and subsequent) paragraphs of the quoted material five more spaces.
- Do not use quotation marks.
- However, place within *double quotation marks* a quotation within a block quotation.
- After the quotation, type the page number of the quotation within parentheses.
- Do not type a period after the closing parenthesis.
- Begin your text with a new paragraph.

Block Quotation	Note
In his powerful explanation of language intervention, Numbskull (2015) asserted: Language intervention is a process of unleashing powerful but painfully hidden but unconsciously active communication potential. The goals of language intervention include transcendental self- actualization, cognitive reorganization, and reconstruction of perceptual–emotive reality. The process of language intervention is mysterious. A successful clinician has an innate ability to solve this mystery. (p. 19) Numbskull's explanation is now a basis for many language treatment programs. Clinicians who despise tiresome objectivity in language treatment have gladly adopted this view.	Alternatively, you may end the quotation with the name, year, and the page number (or numbers) in parentheses: Several experts believe that language intervention is the unleashing of communication potential. Consider the following for instance: Language intervention is a process of unleashing powerful but painfully hidden but unconsciously active communication potential. The goals of language intervention include transcendental self- actualization, cognitive reorganization, and reconstruction of perceptual–emotive reality. The process of language intervention is mysterious. A successful clinician has an innate ability to solve this mystery. (Numbskull, 2015, p. 19) Numbskull's explanation is now a basis for . . .

A.2.32b. Arrange Quotations as a *Block* When They Have 40 Words or More

Quotation of More Than 40 Words	Arrange It Properly
Dumdoom (1992) has stated that "the root cause of stuttering is lack of a shining self-image. That fluent speech is a function of self-image that throws bright light into the eyes of the listener is well established. Therefore, to induce fluency in persons who stutter, we must find ways of polishing their self-image, so it begins to shine again" (pp. 35–36). All clinicians should consider this powerful explanation of stuttering in planning treatment for their clients. Treatment based on this explanation will undoubtedly solve the nagging problem of maintaining fluency.	

A.2.33a. Show Correctly the Changes in Quotations

- When you omit words from a sentence within a quotation, insert an ellipsis mark (three dots) with a space before and after each dot (e.g., mark . . .).
- When you omit words between sentences, insert a space after the period and then insert the three dots of the ellipsis; the three dots of the ellipsis are separated by a space, and there is a space after the ellipsis (e.g., mark. . . .).
- Do not insert ellipses marks at the beginning and end of a quotation, even when it begins or ends in midsentence.
- If you insert words into a quotation, enclose them within brackets.
- Italicize the words *you* emphasize in the quotation that were not emphasized in the original; next to the italicized word, type the words [emphasis added] within brackets.
- Add quotation marks, author name, year of publication, and the page number as shown in the examples.

Changed Quotation	Note
Bluff has stated that "stuttering cannot be measured by . . . merely counting dysfluencies" (2005, p. 58).	Omitted words within a sentence indicated: *by . . . merely* (three dots [ellipsis] with space in between each dot)
"Stuttering and dysfluencies are not to be confused. . . . Stuttering is more than mere dysfluencies" (Bluff, 2005, p. 59).	Omitted words between sentences indicated by a period and three dots: *confused. . . . Stuttering* (the dots after the period are each separated by one space)
According to Bluff, "stuttering is not a speech problem. There is no need to treat it as a communication disorder. It [stuttering] is a problem of cognitive dissonance" (2005, p. 67).	A word may be inserted into a quotation to make the reference clear. The inserted word or words are bracketed: It [stuttering] in this example.
Bluff's extraordinary claim is that "stuttering treatment should involve *cognitive rehabilitation*" [emphasis added] (2005, p. 68).	One or more words in the quotation may be italicized to add emphasis. Note that all quotations need the author's name, year of publication, and the page number or numbers with p. or pp. as its abbreviation.

A.2.33b. Show Correctly the Changes in Quotations

Changed Quotation	Rewrite Correctly
Snuff has stated that "Voice disorders are not only a product of various medical pathologies (words omitted) but also a product of certain life styles. Therefore, clinicians should take a careful and detailed history of the client (words omitted at the end of the sentence). Information obtained through history is invaluable in planning treatment for voice clients (the last three words added). They (the clinicians: *added words*) should not hesitate to probe the *client's life style*" (the last three words italicized to add emphasis; not in the original) (2002, p. 50). *Hint:* More than 40 words!	

A.2.34a. Quote Correctly the Sources on the Internet

- Quoting internet sources with no print editions can be challenging partly because the sources tend to change in both accessibility and content.
- The author, the date, and the page numbers of materials published online may be unclear.
- Reliability and validity of the materials posted may be difficult to assess.
- It is prudent to limit quotes from blogs, wikis, and other such unstable and potentially unreliable sources on the internet unless such sources are a topic of research or discussion.

Quote Correctly	Note
Johns (2015) stated that "the frequency of dysfluencies is more important than their type" (para. 7).	When the page numbers are not available, give the paragraph number if possible (para., abbreviated).
In his study, Williams (2008) claimed that "a genetic basis of child language disorders will soon be discovered" (Introductory section, para. 4).	If no continuous paragraph or page numbers are available for the entire article, specify the section heading and the paragraph number (manually counted) under the heading.
The authors suggested that "early intervention for language disorders is the best means of promoting later academic success" (Boss & Best, 2016, "Promoting Academic Success," para. 2).	When no page or paragraph numbers for the entire article are available, and the heading is too long, abbreviate the heading. In this example, the heading was "Promoting Academic Success Through Early Language Intervention in Children From Low Socioeconomic Backgrounds in Urban Settings." You will have to omit the paragraph number if it is not possible to determine.

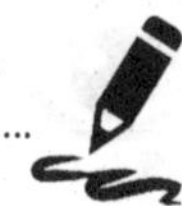

A.2.34b. Quote Correctly the Sources on the Internet

Quote	Write Correctly
Thomas wrote that "the voice disorders need a more valid system of classification" Year: 2015; no page numbers Paragraph, 3	
In his study, James concluded that "autism spectrum disorder is not caused by vaccinations of any kind" Year: 2017 No page number Section heading: Discussion Paragraph, 7 under that section	
The authors suggested that "nodules are better treated with vocal behavior modification" Year: 2013 Authors: Ram and Jam No page number Paragraph 2 Full title: Treating vocal nodules and the attending voice disorders in professional singers and teachers a large urban setting.	

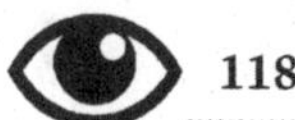

Precision in the Use of Scientific Terms

A.2.35a. Use the Terms Ending in *-ology* Correctly

A few terms that end with *ology* are frequently misused even in scholarly and clinical writing. Ths suffix *-ology* denotes a study of something or a branch of learning. Therefore, *phonology group*, *phonology disorder*, and *impaired morphology* imply that the writer or speaker is careless in using technical terms.

Incorrect	Correct	Note
The child had a disordered morphology.	The child does not produce certain morphological features.	*Disordered morphology* means chaotic study of morphological aspects of language!
The disordered phonology was a major clinical concern.	The phonological disorder was a major clinical concern.	Is the study of phonological aspects of language disordered?
She described the child's phonology.	She described the child's phonological skills.	Did the child produce a branch of learning called phonology?
We had two groups in the study: A phonology disorder group and a group with typical speech.	We had two groups in the study: a group of children with phonological disorders and a group of children without such disorders.	*Disordered phonology* is a frequent mistake in the writings of speech-language pathologists.
Because of his cancer, his physiology is disordered.	Because of his cancer, his physiological system is upset.	These atypical mistakes highlight the inappropriateness of *disordered phonology* and *impaired morphology*. State precisely what is observed to be wrong or impaired.
A brain tumor implies disordered neurology.	A brain tumor implies a neurological disorder (disease).	
Her psychology is off.	Her emotional state is disturbed.	

Precision in the Use of Scientific Terms

A.2.35b. Use the Terms Ending in *-ology* Correctly

Incorrect	Write Correctly
The client has a disturbed morphology.	
The child's morphology should be targeted for treatment.	
The assessment results show that the child's phonology is disordered.	
A good description of a client's phonology is essential before starting phonological treatment.	
Her biology is impaired. *Hint:* Specify a biological system.	
His psychology is disturbed. *Hint:* Specify a psychological disturbance.	
The patient with aphasia has impaired neurology. *Hint:* Neurological impairments	

A.2.36a. Use Certain Terms Ending in *-ics* Correctly

Certain terms that end with *-ics* mean the study of something. Such terms should be used to refer only to a study of something, body of knowledge, discipline, or branch of learning. Such terms as *impaired semantics* or *disordered pragmatics* are examples of careless usage of technical terms and imply ironically that the study itself is impaired or disordered.

<table>
<tr><th>Incorrect</th><th>Correct</th><th>Note</th></tr>
<tr><td>His semantics is impaired.</td><td>His understanding of meaning (semantic features) is impaired.

His productions suggest impaired semantic skills.</td><td>Semantics is the study of meaning in language; it cannot be impaired.</td></tr>
<tr><td>Her semantics needs treatment.</td><td>Her semantic features are a treatment goal.</td><td>She does not study meaning in language.</td></tr>
<tr><td>The client's pragmatics needs help.</td><td>The client's pragmatic skills need treatment.</td><td>Does the client's study of language use need help?</td></tr>
<tr><td>The impaired pragmatics requires advanced training.</td><td>The impaired pragmatic language skills require advanced training.</td><td>Does the study of pragmatic aspects of language require advanced training?</td></tr>
<tr><td>The child's linguistics is impaired.</td><td>The child's language performance is impaired.</td><td rowspan="2">These atypical mistakes point out the inappropriateness of such terms as impaired semantics and disordered pragmatics.</td></tr>
<tr><td>Studies have shown that disordered genetics may partly be responsible for stuttering that runs in families.</td><td>Studies have shown that genetic factors may partly be responsible for stuttering that runs in families.</td></tr>
</table>

A.2.36b. Use Certain Terms Ending in *-ics* Correctly

Incorrect	Write Correctly
Her semantics is difficult to analyze.	
Semantics was one of the treatment goals.	
His use of pragmatics is questionable.	
Her pragmatics should be a treatment target.	
The child's linguistics is impaired.	
The man's genetics is faulty.	

Use of Fresh Language

A.2.37a. Avoid Clichés

- Clichés are overused, dull, and stale expressions; they include most idioms.
- Replace clichés and idioms with direct and fresh expressions.

Cliché	Simple and Direct	Note
We do not have many *tried-and-true* treatment techniques.	We do not have many proven treatment techniques.	The word *proven* is more acceptable for this kind of writing.
Though he recently had a stroke, the patient was *fit as a fiddle*.	Though he recently had a stroke, the patient was in good health.	An everyday term is more appropriate than the cliché.
Treating persons with laryngectomy is not her *cup of tea*.	1. She does not enjoy treating persons with laryngectomy. 2. She is not trained in treating persons who have had laryngectomy.	Some clichés mask multiple meanings.
In *this day and age*, the clinician needs to have computer skills.	The clinician needs to have computer skills.	

A.2.38a. Avoid Colloquial or Informal Expressions

- Avoid such expressions in scientific and professional writing.
- Use your judgment in including them in informal and general writing.

Informal	Formal	Note
If the client *can't* imitate, I will use the shaping method.	If the client *cannot* imitate, I will use the shaping method.	Avoid contractions in formal and scientific writing.
Continuous reinforcement *won't* be used.	Continuous reinforcement *will not* be used.	
The researcher *felt* that the procedure was effective.	The researcher *thought* that the procedure was effective.	Avoid such subjective terms as *felt* unless the reference is to feelings.
The clinician *came up* with a dysphagia assessment procedure.	The clinician *developed* a dysphagia assessment procedure.	

Use of Fresh Language

A.2.37b. Avoid Clichés

Cliché	Write in Simple and Direct Words
The child is bored to tears with therapy.	
The initial progress gave the client a shot in the arm.	
The child who stutters is sick and tired of teasing from her friends.	
In promoting maintenance, I will leave no stone unturned.	
My treatment plan was off track.	

A.2.38b. Avoid Colloquial or Informal Expressions

Informal	Formal
The client just wouldn't imitate the modeled stimulus.	
The clinician hadn't prepared the stimulus materials.	
I feel that the client's hoarseness of voice is due to vocal nodules.	
The clinician cooked up a novel method of evoking the /r/.	

A.3. Commonly Misused Words and Phrases

Avoid the common mistakes of misusing words that sound similar but have different meanings.

A.3.1a. *Accept* and *Except*

Accept means to receive something offered; *except* means with the exclusion of (something or someone). Erroneous substitution of *except* for *accept* is common.

Incorrect	Correct	Note
I *except* your kind offer.	I *accept* your kind offer.	The incorrect expressions do not make sense. The incorrect expression may be interpreted to mean the opposite of what is intended.
She *excepted* our gift.	She *accepted* our gift.	
I was the only one *accepted* from the regulation.	I was the only one *excepted* from the regulation.	
All were admitted into the bar, *accept* me.	All were admitted into the bar, *except* me.	
I will *except* all conditions *accept* the first.	I will *accept* all conditions *except* the first.	

A.3.2a. *Affect* and *Effect*

Generally, use *affect* as a verb and *effect* as a noun. **Exceptions:** Use *effect* (or the term *to effect*) always as a verb or verb phrase when the meaning is *to cause a change* or *create an effect* (e.g., *Education is intended to effect changes in thinking*); use *affect* as a noun when it refers to an emotional state (e.g., *When he lost the bet, his affect changed*).

Incorrect	Correct
Many researchers have studied the masking noise *affect* on stuttering.	Many researchers have studied the masking noise *effect* on stuttering.
She studied the treatment *affects*.	She studied the treatment *effects*.
The treatment *effected* the behavior.	The treatment *affected* the behavior.
How did the variable *effect* the outcome?	How did the variable *affect* the outcome?
The clinician's goal is *to affect* changes in the client's communication skills.	The clinician's goal is to *effect* changes in the client's communication skills.
The clinician could not *affect* changes in the client's naming skills.	The clinician could not *effect* changes in the client's naming skills.

A.3.1b. *Accept* and *Except*

Incorrect	Write Correctly
I am pleased to except your job offer.	
He did not except our offer of assistance.	
Everyone got in, accept John.	
The faculty excepted all applicants, accept one.	
Scientists have excepted these theories, accept perhaps the first.	

A.3.2b. *Affect* and *Effect*

Incorrect	Write Correctly
The affect of environmental deprivation on language acquisition is significant.	
This study on the affect of aphasia treatment was poorly designed.	
Modeling effected the target response.	
To affect changes in clients' behaviors, the clinician needs strong treatment programs.	
How does the parental dysfluency rate effect the child's stuttering?	
In spite of her excellent efforts, the clinician could not affect changes in the patient's cognitive skills.	*Hint: to cause changes* (the exceptional case).

A.3.3a. *Alternate* and *Alternative*

Alternate means different events occurring or succeeding by turns; to alternate is to shift from one to the other. *Alternative* suggests a choice between two possibilities.

Incorrect	Correct	Note
We will use the two *alternative* treatments to see if one is more effective than the other.	We will *alternate* the two treatments to see if one is better than the other.	Clinician shifts from one treatment to the other; both are offered in different sessions.
The appliance uses *alternative* current.	The appliance uses *alternating* current.	Current reverses its direction at regular intervals.
I will take the *alternate* route.	I will take the *alternative* route.	The person chose the other route.
The only *alternate* to treatment is continued stuttering.	The only a*lternative* to treatment is continued stuttering.	The statement says there is only one choice.

A.3.4a. *Allusion* and *Illusion*

Use *illusion* to refer to an unreal image and *allusion* to suggest an indirect reference.

Incorrect	Correct
She made an *illusion* to the new theory of voice production.	She made an *allusion* to the new theory of voice production. [*Better:* She alluded to]
The ghost he thought he saw was merely an *allusion.*	The ghost he thought he saw was merely an *illusion.*

A.3.5a. *And/Or*

Avoid a*nd/or* because the meaning could be ambiguous. Rewrite the sentence.

Incorrect	Correct
Pictures *and/or* objects will be used to evoke the target behaviors.	Pictures, objects, *or both* will be used to evoke the target behaviors.
Speech-language pathologists *and/or* psychologists may assess persons with dementia.	Speech-language pathologists, psychologists, *or both* may assess persons with dementia.

A.3.3b. *Alternate* and *Alternative*

Incorrect	Write Correctly
It leaves me with no alternate.	
You can alternative the two probe procedures.	
We will alternatively use auditory comprehension and speech production to see which one is more effective.	
The alternate to a college education is a low-paying job.	

A.3.4b. *Allusion* and *Illusion*

Incorrect	Write Correctly
He made an illusion to an emerging trend in the treatment of dysarthria.	
The treatment effects reported in the study were merely an allusion.	

A.3.5b. *And/Or*

Incorrect	Write Correctly
The father and/or the mother of the client will be trained in response maintenance.	
Language disorders and/or phonological disorders may coexist with stuttering.	

A.3.6a. *Baseline* and *Baserate*

- Use *baseline* only as a noun.
- Use *baserate* as a verb or as a noun.
- Note that the words *baserate* and *baseline* are single words (not written as *base rate* or *base line*).

Incorrect	Correct	Note
Before starting treatment, the clinician should *baseline* target behaviors.	Before starting treatment, the clinician should establish *baselines* of target behaviors.	*Baselines* incorrectly used as a verb and correctly used as a noun.
I *baselined* the target responses. I will *baseline* sound productions.	I will establish *baselines* of target responses. I will *baserate* sound productions.	*Baseline* incorrectly used as a verb and correctly substituted with *baserate. Baserate* correctly used as a noun.

A.3.7a. *Effect* and *Impact*

- In scientific writing, prefer the term *effect* to currently popular *impact*; your "treatment makes an impact" only when the treatment collides your clients and gets stuck to them.
- *Impact* is striking of one body against the other (e.g., *the man who jumped from the fifth floor died of injuries caused by the impact).*
- *Impact* also means *to pack firmly (e.g., the wax in the client's ear was impacted*).

Inaccurate	Accurate	Note
Modeling has an *impact* on the child's productions.	Modeling has an *effect* on the child's productions.	Modeling does not strike or firmly pack the client's productions.
This treatment is known to have an *impact.*	This treatment is known to have an *effect.*	The traditional word does fine.
The *impact* of poverty on language acquisition needs additional research.	The *effect* of poverty on language acquisition needs additional research.	

A.3.6b. *Baseline* and *Baserate*

Incorrect	Write Correctly
All target behaviors should be baselined before starting treatment.	
I first baselined turn taking in conversation.	
I will baseline morphological productions.	1. Correct noun form: 2. Correct verb form:

A.3.7b. *Effect* and *Impact*

Inaccurate	Write More Accurately
Slow rate of speech has a profound impact on stuttering.	
Several investigators have analyzed the impact of noise on speech.	
The impact of treatment was negligible.	

A.3.8a. *Elicit* and *Evoke*

- Note that a stimulus (e.g., a tap on the knee) *elicits* a reflexive response (e.g., a knee-jerk reflex), and a different stimulus (e.g., a picture) *evokes* a voluntary response (e.g., a name from a person with aphasia).
- In natural settings or in treatment sessions, speech-language responses, being voluntary, are not *elicited* but are *evoked.*
- Prefer the word *evoke* to imply the action of stimulating speech and language responses in assessment or treatment sessions.

Less Accurate	More Accurate	Note
I will *elicit* a language sample from the child.	I will *evoke* a language sample from the child.	Technically, reflexive responses are *elicited*, and voluntary responses are *evoked.* Pupil dilation is elicited, but speech and language productions are evoked.
A flash of light will *evoke* pupil dilation.	A flash of light will *elicit* pupil dilation.	
Pavlov *evoked* the salivary reflex by placing meat powder in the dog's mouth.	Pavlov *elicited* the salivary reflex by placing meat powder in the dog's mouth.	
By reinforcing them, Skinner *elicited* and increased the bar-pressing responses in rats.	By reinforcing them, Skinner *evoked* and increased the bar-pressing responses in rats.	

A.3.9a. *Elicit* and *Illicit*

- Because of an especially troublesome confusion, some students try to *illicit target responses.*
- Note that *illicit* is not a verb, it is an adjective (but a supervisor with no sense of humor may pull out handcuffs!).

Incorrect	Correct	Note
Pictures will be used to *illicit* the phoneme.	Pictures will be used to *evoke* the phoneme.	The less accurate *elicit* is preferable to the illegal *illicit.*
I will teach the mother to *illicit* the target behaviors at home.	I will teach the mother to *evoke* the target behaviors at home.	

A.3.8b. *Elicit* and *Evoke*

Less Accurate	Write More Accurately
Pavlov evoked the salivary reflex.	
Skinner elicited the bar-press response.	
There are many procedures to elicit the production of /s/.	
I will evoke the psychogalvanic reflex.	
I know a few methods of evoking the swallow reflex.	

A.3.9b. *Elicit* and *Illicit*

Incorrect	Write Correctly
She illicited single-word responses from her client.	
I will demonstrate in front of a mirror to illicit /k/.	
I will use pictures to illicit naming responses from my patient with aphasia.	

Note: There is no such word as *illicited.*

A.3.10a. *Farther* and *Further*

Use *farther* to refer to distance. Use *further* to refer to time or quantity.

Incorrect	Correct
She walked *further* than any person.	She walked *farther* than any person.
I sent the parents a *farther* notice of an IEP meeting.	I sent the parents a *further* notice of an IEP meeting.
Farthermore, the client was often late.	*Furthermore*, the client was often late.

A.3.11a. *Focus* and *Analysis*

- Note that *focus* is another fancy term whose popularity is ever escalating.
- In scientific writing, substitute this term with more appropriate terms, including *study* or *analysis*.

<table>
<tr><th>Vague</th><th>More Precise</th><th>Note</th></tr>
<tr><td>In her lecture, she focused on the principles of aerobic dancing.</td><td>In her lecture, she elaborated the principles of aerobic dancing.</td><td>The term focus does not say what the lecturer did.</td></tr>
<tr><td>To prevent heart diseases, scientists are focusing on people's dietary habits.</td><td>To prevent heart diseases, scientists are studying people's dietary habits.</td><td rowspan="2">Just focusing on a problem may not help analyze it or solve it.</td></tr>
<tr><td>In solving the crime problem, investigators have focused on family dynamics.</td><td>In solving the crime problem, investigators have analyzed family dynamics.</td></tr>
</table>

A.3.10b. *Farther* and *Further*

Incorrect	Write Correctly
New York is further than you think.	
After establishing the target behaviors, the clinician should do farther work on maintenance.	
I will study the subject farther.	

A.3.11b. *Focus* and *Analysis*

Vague	Write More Precisely
Because I am getting poor grades, I need to focus on my study skills.	
The instructor focused on some difficult theories.	
The researchers now focus on the genetic bases of hearing loss.	

A.3.12a. *Incidence* and *Prevalence*

- *Incidence* is the future occurrence of an event in a population. (*How many fluently speaking children will begin to stutter in a 12-month period?*)
- *Prevalence* is the number of persons affected by something; you take a head count. (*How many children in the school district currently have a hearing loss?*)

Incorrect	Correct	Note
The *incidence* of stuttering in the U.S. population is about 2 million.	The *incidence* of stuttering in the population is about 1%. The prevalence of stuttering in the country is about 2 million.	Incidence of stuttering refers to the number of typically fluent people who will begin to stutter in a 12-month period.
The *prevalence* of hearing loss is about 10%.	The *prevalence* of hearing loss in Fresno is about 1,100 children. The *incidence* of hearing loss is about 10%.	Prevalence refers to the total number of persons who already have a characteristic or a disorder.

A.3.13a. *Inter-* and *Intra-*

Inter- means *between* or *among*. *Intra-* means *within*.

Incorrect	Correct	Note
The *intraobserver* reliability index is based on the observations of two graduate students.	The *intraobserver* reliability index is based on two observations of the same graduate student.	To determine *intraobserver* reliability, the same person should repeat observations.
The *interobserver* reliability index is based on the experimenter's two observations.	The *interobserver* reliability index is based on the observations of the experimenter and an outside expert.	To determine *interobserver* reliability, two or more persons should observe the same event.
I will take an *intrastate* highway to cross the state boundary.	I will take an *interstate* highway to cross the state boundary.	An *interstate* highway runs across states.
Motivation is an *interpersonal* variable.	Motivation is an *intrapersonal* variable.	Motivation is a within-person factor.

A.3.12b. *Incidence* and *Prevalence*

Incorrect	Write Correctly
The incidence of strokes in the country is about 500,000.	
The prevalence of language disorders in the school-age children in the city is 10%.	

A.3.13b. *Inter-* and *Intra-*

Incorrect	Correct
I will correlate my measures of dysfluencies with those of another clinician to establish the intraobserver reliability.	
The experimenter correlated two of her observations to establish the interobserver reliability index.	
At least two observers are needed to calculate an intraobserver reliability index.	
The same observer has to make at least two observations to calculate an interobserver reliability index.	

A.3.14a. *Latter* and *Later*

- *Latter* is the second of the two things just mentioned (*former* is the first of the two).
- *Later* refers to time: it refers to something done after another activity or time period.

Incorrect	Correct	Note
Teach the skills first, and work on maintenance *latter.*	Teach the skills first, and work on maintenance *later.*	Your work on maintenance comes later in time.
Your training criterion may be 80% or 90% correct; the *later* requires more training.	Your training criterion may be 80% or 90% correct; the *latter* requires more training.	The latter refers to the second of the two criteria mentioned (90%). The term helps avoid repetition of an element.

A.3.15a. *Proof* and *Support*

- The terms *proof, proved,* or *disproved* are overstatements in science.
- Prefer the words *support, evidence, confirm,* and so forth, as shown in the examples.

<table>
<tr><th>Less Accurate</th><th>More Accurate</th><th>Note</th></tr>
<tr><td>My data prove that there is a gene for grammar.</td><td>My data support the hypothesis that there is a gene for grammar.</td><td rowspan="2">Take note of other substitutes for proof.</td></tr>
<tr><td>These observations prove that the treatment was effective.</td><td>These observations suggest that the treatment was effective.</td></tr>
<tr><td>Johnson proved that the Native Americans do not stutter.</td><td>Johnson claimed that the Native Americans do not stutter.</td><td rowspan="2">The word claimed suggests skepticism about the hypothesis.</td></tr>
<tr><td>More recent studies have disproved Johnson's claim.</td><td>More recent studies have contradicted Johnson's claim.</td></tr>
<tr><td>The data prove the stated hypotheses.</td><td>The data confirm the stated hypotheses.</td><td>A hypothesis is confirmed, not proven.</td></tr>
</table>

A.3.14.b. *Latter* and *Later*

Incorrect	Correct
I am busy now; I will do it latter.	
First, I will teach; latter I will probe.	
Both treatment and counseling are essential; the later requires additional clinical skills.	
I took courses on biology and physics; I liked the former but hated the later.	

A.3.15b. *Proof* and *Support*

Less Accurate	Write More Accurately
The linguists have proved that there is an innate language acquisition device.	
My data prove that the hypothesis is invalid.	
Becker proved that all children are born with universal grammar.	
Recent research disproves her claim.	

A.3.16a. *Secondly* and *Thirdly*

- Avoid those terms.
- Write: *First, Second, Third,* and so forth.

Not Preferred	Preferred	Note
First, I will assess the client. *Secondly,* I will select the target behaviors. *Thirdly,* I will prepare the stimulus materials.	*First,* I will assess the client. *Second,* I will select the target behaviors. *Third,* I will prepare the stimulus materials.	Some write *firstly,* but it is worse than *secondly* and *thirdly.*

A.3.17a. *Since* and *Because*

- *Since* suggests a temporal sequence of events from a specified time, as in *Since the introduction of digital technology, hearing aids have been more acceptable than before.*
- *Because* suggests causation, as in *Because the man stuttered, he did not ask questions.*

Incorrect or Less Precise	Correct	Note
Since the stimulus pictures are ambiguous, the responses are not certain.	*Because* the stimulus pictures are ambiguous, the responses are not certain.	Ambiguous pictures cause uncertain responses.

A.3.18a. *There* and *Their*

There suggests location, and *their* suggests group possession.

Incorrect	Correct	Note
This is *there* house.	This is *their* house.	
Their is the book you wanted.	*There* is the book you wanted.	
Was *their* a party tonight?	Was *there* a party tonight?	
How is *there* health?	How is *their* health?	

A.3.16b. *Secondly* and *Thirdly*

Not Preferred	Preferred
First, I will instruct the client. Secondly, I will place the headphones on the client. Thirdly, I will begin hearing testing.	

A.3.17b. *Since* and *Because*

Incorrect or Inaccurate	Write Correctly
Since the auditory discrimination procedure was not effective, I shifted to production training.	
Since the child is not cooperative, automatic audiologic assessment procedures are necessary.	

A.3.18b. *There* and *Their*

Incorrect	Write Correctly
That was once there haunt.	
Their is what you need.	
I thought their was going to be a quiz today.	
How is there new baby?	

Note to Student Writers

Examples on the previous pages represent only a small number of commonly misused words and phrases. Use this page to write down additional examples of such words and phrases. Practice correct usage of those words and phrases.

Misused Words	Correct Usage

Note: Many books on writing contain sections on word usage.

PART B

Scientific Writing

B.1. Introduction to Scientific Writing

Printed Notes	Class Notes

Scientific writing is

- related to data, research, or theory
- direct
- precise
- objective
- organized according to an accepted format

Scientific journals have their specific formats. Journals like those of the American Speech-Language-Hearing Association (ASHA) use a format that is based on the *Publication Manual of the American Psychological Association* (7th ed., 2020) (APA Manual).

However, please take note that ASHA journals do not strictly follow the APA Manual in all respects. Certain aspects of article design including heading styles and reference citations of ASHA may vary from the APA style.

All writing is designed for an audience. In addition, scientific and professional writing is designed for an agency or a source of publication. For example, a research paper may be designed according to the format prescribed by a journal to which it is submitted. A grant proposal, on the other hand, may be designed according to the guidelines of a government agency or a private foundation.

Undergraduate and graduate students write term papers. Advanced graduate students may write research papers, theses, and dissertations. In completing their writing projects, students should follow a prescribed format. The instructor of a course, the university's graduate school, or the policy of the academic department may dictate the format.

Students should find out the accepted or prescribed format and write accordingly. Throughout this part on scientific writing, the APA style is used for illustration. Certain unique features of the ASHA journals are highlighted.

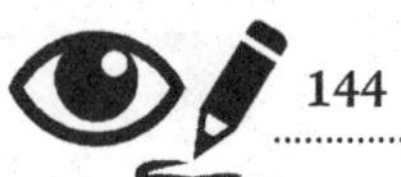

Printed Notes	Class Notes

There always are reasons to deviate from a particular style. You should ascertain from your instructor the acceptable deviations from the prescribed style. Potential or recommended deviations from the APA Manual guidelines are specified in this section.

Please note that most books do not fully conform to the APA style in its headings, paragraph indentations, margins, the use of italics and underlining, and so forth. A coursebook, such as this one, has a unique format as you can see. General design features that are appropriate for an article or a term paper may not be appropriate for a book. Each publishing company uses its own style in designing books. For aesthetic reasons, headings, paragraph styles, and so forth, often are uniquely designed for each book. Therefore, students should not look at book designs, including the design of this book, to understand the APA style.

B.2. Terms for Writing Without Bias

Printed Notes	Class Notes

An important writing skill is to avoid bias. Writing should be free from biases related to race, ethnicity, age, disability, socioeconomic status, sexual orientation, gender, and gender identity. Pronouns that suggest male dominance, prejudicial references to gender identity and sexual orientation, and negative connotations about disabilities and aging should be avoided. Scientific and clinical writing should be free from stereotypic and prejudicial language about people with limited income, education, and racial and cultural diversity. Persons with disorders and diseases should be described in respectful terms. Clinical and nonclinical groups recruited for research should be described in language that does not suggest negative evaluation. Language that suggests biases may be used, as done in the following pages, only to point out their inappropriateness and suggest more appropriate bias-free writing samples.

In research reports, references to gender, gender identity, sexual orientation, disability, socioeconomic status, and ethnic or racial background may be made when a knowledge of such factors is essential to understand the results of a piece of research. The selected terms related to such factors should be

- nonevaluative, nonoffensive, and neutral
- those the groups use to refer to themselves

Note that biases show up not just in scientific writing but in all kinds of writing, everyday speech, and behavior in general. Scientists and clinicians do not merely avoid biased writing; they learn anti-racist and antidiscriminatory patterns of verbal and nonverbal behaviors. Their actions show an appreciation of cultural diversity and a commitment to equality and justice. Bias-free writing is one of the desirable patterns of behavior.

The following pages in this section give examples of bias-free writing and opportunities to practice it. Before practicing bias-free writing, however, it is essential to understand various terms that should be used correctly. Therefore, to complete the practice pages, it is essential to read the definitions of the following terms.

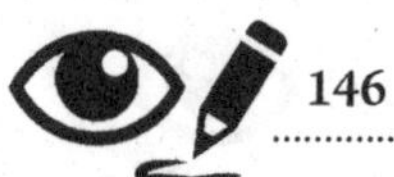

Printed Notes	Class Notes

Ableism: Prejudice against people with physical disabilities; belief that able-bodied people are superior to people with disability.

Adultism: Discounting or discriminating against children and adolescents; a form of ageism.

African: People living in Africa; not a synonym for *African American*; specificity is preferred (e.g., *Nigerian*, *Ethiopian*, or if appropriate, *Nigerian American, Ethiopian American*).

African American: People of African background or ancestry who live in the United States; *Black* is an accepted alternative; *Afro-American* is outdated; *Negro* is offensive.

Aged: An outdated term for older persons.

Ageism: Stereotyping and discriminating against persons who are old; similar to *racism*.

Ageist: Similar to *racist*; the practice of, or the one who practices, ageism.

Agender: Lack of gender or gender neutral; may or may not be asexual; for pronouns, ask the person.

Asexual: A person who experiences little or no sexual and romantic attraction toward any person.

Asian American: Person of Asian background or ancestry living in the United States; not a synonym for the *Asian* who lives in Asia; specificity is preferred (e.g., *Chinese American*, *Sri Lankan American*, *Korean American*, *Indian American*, etc.).

Audism: Prejudice against people with hearing loss; belief that people with typical hearing are superior to those with hearing loss.

Binary: Either male or female in the gender-related literature.

Bisexual: A person whose sexual and romantic attraction may extend to persons of the same gender or those of other genders.

Black or White people: The only two groups of people who may be identified by their skin color; people of any other color not to be identified in this manner (e.g., do not write *brown people*).

Caucasian: An outdated term for the *White* or the *White European*; not to be used.

Chicana/Chicano: Persons of Mexican origin or ancestry; gendered; also may be called Hispanics, but not all Hispanics are Chicana/o.

Printed Notes	Class Notes

Cisgender: A person whose gender identity and sexual orientation are consistent with the sex assigned at birth; most people are *cismale* or *cisfemale.*

Cross-dresser: A person who partially or fully dresses like a person belonging to a gender other than what was assigned at birth; does not imply a particular sexual orientation; replaces *transvestite.*

Deaf: A preferred, capitalized term by those who belong to the Deaf culture and use a variety of sign languages.

Demisexual: A person who is not sexually attracted to someone unless also emotionally attracted or bonded.

Elderly: An outdated term for the older person.

Ethnicity: Shared language, culture, beliefs, and behavior patterns that help identify a group of people; not a synonym of *race.*

Gay men: Persons who are sexually and romantically attracted to individuals of the same sex and gender.

Gender: Feelings and behaviors a society or culture associates with the biological sex of a person; a social identity construct.

Gender-affirming surgery: Surgical modification of a person's body to make it consistent with that person's gender identity; also called *gender-confirming* or *sex reassignment* surgery; not all transgender people will have undergone this surgery; replaces *sex change operation*, a term not to be used.

Gender binary: The concept that gender can only be female or male and should behave as society expects; prejudicial term.

Gender diversity: Varied gender identities; an umbrella term that includes different gender identities; some may prefer this to *gender nonbinary* or *gender nonconforming.*

Gender dysphoria: Distress caused by an incongruence between a person's felt or expressed gender and the social role expected on the basis of sex assigned at birth. A controversial *Diagnostic and Statistical Manual of Mental Disorders* (5th ed.; *DSM-5*) psychiatric diagnostic term; replaces *gender identity disorder.*

Gender expression: Gender-related overt behaviors including appearance (e.g., clothing and hairstyle), speech, voice, personal pronoun usage, and general behavior. Gender expression and gender identity may or may not be identical.

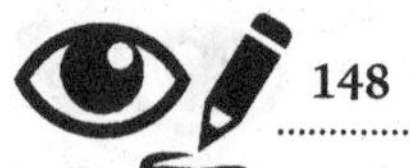

Printed Notes	Class Notes

Gender-fluid: Variable gender identity across time.

Gender identity: Self-description of one's gender and pronoun and a pattern of behavior consistent with that description; deeply felt feelings about one's sense of being a person of certain gender, no fixed gender, or no gender (agender); may be binary (girl, boy, man, woman) or nonbinary (genderqueer, gender fluid, gender nonconforming, transgender, two-spirit, etc.); may be consistent with sex assigned at birth or at variance.

Gender nonconforming: Persons whose gender-related behaviors are inconsistent with social expectations; not a synonym for *transgender*.

Genderqueer: Persons whose gender expressions are somewhere in between the male–female identity, totally outside of male–female identities, or with their own unique identities; not a synonym for *transgender*, although may be used as an umbrella term for varied gender identities.

Hearing loss: Hearing acuity reduced to varying degrees; preferable to *hearing impairment*.

Heterosexism: A belief that heterosexual behavior is normal; refers to prejudice and discriminatory behavior toward those with diverse sexual orientation.

Hispanic: Geographically dispersed and culturally varied people of Spanish-language background; not a race; preferable to be specific (e.g., *Mexican American*, *Cuban American*, *Chilean American*).

Homoprejudice: Prejudicial beliefs and behaviors toward lesbians and gay men; also called *homonegativity* and *homophobia*.

Homosexuality: Sexual attraction felt toward persons of the same sex and gender; an outdated and prejudicial term because of the past legal sanctions and implications of pathology.

Identity-first language: Describing disability by starting with the disability itself; person comes next (e.g., *Deaf person*, not the *person who is deaf*; *autistic person*, not *the person with autism*); to be used only when the persons in question prefer it as a matter of personal and sociocultural pride; see *Person-first language*.

Printed Notes	Class Notes

Intellectual disability: Persons with deficits in reasoning, abstract thinking, and academic learning; with deficits in such adaptive functions as personal independence and social responsibility; observed during the developmental period; replaces the term *mental retardation*.

Intersex: Anatomic and biological (e.g., chromosomal patterns) sex characteristics that do not permit a binary classification of male or female; ambiguity may be present at birth or may emerge later, often at puberty.

Latin@: People of Latin American ancestry; varied pronunciation including /lətinaʊ/; another gender-neutral term like *Latinx*.

Latino/Latina: Gendered terms for the people of Latin American (including Brazilian) origin or ancestry; also spelled Latina/o or Latino/a; not a synonym for *Hispanic*; specificity is preferred (e.g., Chilean, Cuban, Bolivian, Mexican); ascertain the personal preference.

Latinx: People of Latin American background or descent; gender neutral because it replaces the gendered *o* or *a*; hence accepted by the LGBTQIA+ communities.

Lesbian: A woman who is sexually and romantically attracted to persons of the same sex and gender.

LGBTQIA+: Lesbian, Gay, Bisexual, Transgender, Queer/Questioning, Intersex, Asexual, and More; an umbrella term, still evolving, for people whose self-identified gender identity and/or sexual orientation are outside of the cisgender heteronormative constructs.

Misogyny: Hatred of women and girls; may lead to violence against them; an extreme form of sexism.

Native American: Indigenous people of the Americas; often used as the native people of the United States or Canada; may be preferable to *American Indian* to avoid confusion with people of India or Indian heritage (*Indian Americans*); specificity is preferred (e.g., *Navajo, Cherokee, Shoshone*); *people* or *nation*, but not *tribe*.

Nonbinary: Refers to a range of gender identities that do not conform to the categorical male/female identity; some may prefer *gender diversity*.

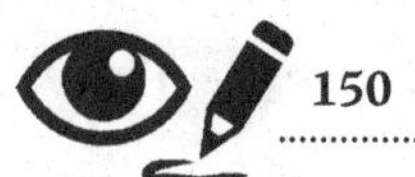

Printed Notes	Class Notes

Oriental: An outdated term for the people of the Eastern hemisphere; pejorative because it has colonial connotations and mainly includes objects considered exotic (e.g., carpets, furniture, decorative art).

Pansexual: Persons who feel sexually attracted to people of all genders and sexes.

People of color: Acceptable alternative to *non-White people*; *underrepresented groups* is acceptable, but *minorities* is not because it is nonspecific and may be inaccurate; in some places, non-Whites may be a majority.

Person-first language: Describing disability by starting with the person (e.g., *person with traumatic brain injury*, *child with language disorder*); see *Identity-first language.*

Queer: Originally used to belittle and demean the community of lesbian, gay, bisexual, and transsexual individuals, now many in the same community have reclaimed the word for their own designation as a matter of pride; not all members of this community may accept the term, so it is essential to ask the person for preference.

Questioning: Individuals who are exploring their gender identity and sexual orientation because of uncertainty.

Race: People who share a set of physical features and consider those features socially and culturally significant; terms that refer to racial differences include the *Aboriginal*, *African American*, *White*, *Asian*, *Native American*, *Pacific Islander*, *Native Hawaiian*, and so forth; capitalized because they are proper nouns; see *Ethnicity*.

Senile: An outdated term for persons with *dementia*.

Sex: Assigned male or female category at the time of birth, based on external anatomy; more biological than the personally and socially constructed *gender identity*, which may or may not align with assigned sex.

Sex assignment at birth: What the birth certificate says about the sex of the individual.

Sexism: Discriminatory behavior toward women and girls; may lead to violence against women and girls; in clinical and scientific writing, inappropriate use of male pronouns and other writing styles perpetuate sexism.

Printed Notes	Class Notes

Sexual orientation: A set of blended emotional, romantic, sexual, affectional, and social behaviors that imply sexual attraction or nonattraction to other persons; part of a person's gender and personal identity; replaces *sexual preference.*

Straight: Persons who are sexually attracted to members of another sex.

Transgender: A person whose gender identity and gender-related behaviors differ from the conventional expectations based on their sex assignment at birth; may or may not have undergone gender-affirming surgery; adjective, not a noun.

Transition: A personal (speech, dress), medical (hormonal, surgical), and legal (name change) process of altering one's sex assigned at birth; replaces *sex change.*

Transprejudice: Discriminatory behavior toward transgender; the same as *transnegativity.*

Transsexual: Persons who have transitioned through medical intervention; an older term; most people prefer to call themselves *transgender.*

Two-spirit: Persons with more than one sexual identity, such as both a male and a female identity; may feel a same-sex or any other-sex attraction; a Native American term.

Underprivileged: People with less money, education, resources, and political power; may be of any race, color, national origin, or ancestry; not a generic term for racial groups or minorities.

Additional Resources

American Psychological Association. (2014). Guidelines for Psychological Practice with Older Adults. *American Psychologist, 69*(1), 34–65. https://doi.org/10.1037/a0035063

American Psychological Association. (2020). *Publication manual of the American Psychological Association* (7th ed.). Author.

Centers for Disease Control and Prevention. (n.d.). *Patient-centered care for transgender people: Recommended practices for healthcare settings.* https://www.cdc.gov/hiv/clinicians/transforming-health/health-care-providers/affirmative-care.html

Taylor, C. (2009). Health and safety issues for Aboriginal transgender/two-spirit people in Manitoba. *Canadian Journal of Aboriginal Community-based HIV/AIDS Research, 2,* 63–84.

B.2.1a. Do Not Overuse the Pronouns *He* and *He or She*

- Do not use *he* as a generic pronoun; use it to refer to an identified male.
- Do not overuse *he or she* to avoid tedious reading; do not write *he/she* or *(s)he*.
- Use the third person plural *they* or *theirs* as a nonbinary single third person pronoun.

Biased or Tedious	Better Alternatives	Note
A client may be reminded that *he* should be punctual.	A client may be reminded that *he or she* should be punctual.	Infrequent use is acceptable, but consider the alternatives.
A person who stutters may withhold *his* opinion.	*Mr. Lopez who* stutters may withhold his opinion.	Appropriate use of *his.*
Animals share only a part of *man's* capacity for communication.	Animals share only a part of *humans'* capacity for communication.	*Humans* or *mankind* may substitute for *man, woman, women, men*
He or she may be asked to respond. Each person gave *his or her* consent.	All *clients* were asked to respond. All *persons* gave consent.	Plurals help avoid the tedious use of *he or she* and *his or her.*
Refer the child to a pediatrician; *he* will diagnose the problem.	Refer the child to a pediatrician *who* will diagnose the problem.	*Who* replaces *he*; gender remains unspecified.
Each child selected a toy *he or she* wanted to play with.	Each child selected a toy *they* wanted to play with.	*They* is gender neutral (nonbinary).
Each client interacted with *his or her* clinician.	Each client interacted with *their* clinician.	Gender-neutral use of *their* as singular.
Busy judges tend to neglect their *wives.*	Busy judges tend to neglect their *spouses.*	Avoids the implication that all judges are male.
A child with intellectual disabilities will be slow in *his* acquisition of language.	A child with intellectual disabilities will be slow in *the* acquisition of language.	Replace the pronoun with an article.
A scientist investigates funding sources available for *her* research.	A scientist investigates funding sources available for research.	Drop the pronoun altogether.

B.2.1b. Do Not Overuse the Pronouns *He* and *He or She*

- Use all the different strategies shown in the previous exemplars.

Biased or Tedious	Suggest Better Alternatives
A client with aphasia may say he is frustrated with speech attempts.	
A client may be asked to rate his fluency.	
Mankind has known about speech problems for a long time.	
Refer the client to a biotechnician. He will fashion a prosthetic device.	
Hearing loss in old age affects a man's social behavior.	
A client should be told at the outset how much he or she will pay for the hearing aids.	*Hint:* nonbinary *they*
A clinician should never evade her ethical responsibility.	*Hint:* gender-neutral *their*
The child should not be thought of merely as a client.	*Hint:* plural noun.
Refer the client to a laryngologist. He will evaluate.	*Hint: who*
Engineers tend to marry women who are artists.	*Hint:* Eliminate the gendered pronoun.

B.2.2a. Use the Appropriate Terms of Gender Identities

- Gender identity is gender self-description.
- Gender identity may be cisfemale, cismale, transgender, or gender nonbinary (which includes gender fluid, genderqueer, gender nonconforming, gender neutral, agender, and other still-evolving terms); *two-spirit* is an Indigenous and Native American term.
- Ascertain and use the individual's self-identified gender identity term or pronoun.
- Some may use alternative pronouns "ze," "xe," "hir," "per," "pe," "ey," and so forth.
- Some permanently medically changed persons may call themselves *transsexual.*
- *Cisgender* person's current gender identity aligns with the sex assignment at birth.
- *Sex assignment* at birth and the current *gender identity* of a person may be different.

Inappropriate	Appropriate	Note
He is transgendered. They are transgender.	He is a transgender person. They are transgender people.	*Transgender* is an adjective, not a noun.
She is a transvestite.	The person is a cross-dresser.	The term *cross-dresser* replaces *transvestite.*
Male-to-female *transformed* person.	Male-to-female *transgender* person.	*Transformed* and *sex- changed* are unacceptable.
She is a female-to-male transgender woman.	*He* is a female-to-male transgender man.	Pronouns should reflect the current gender identity.
We recruited 20 *typical* males and 20 *typical* females.	We recruited 20 *cisgender* males and 20 *cisgender* females.	Avoid terms like *typical* and *normal* to refer to sexual identity.
Some of the participants were *neither male nor female.*	Some of the participants were gender *nonbinary.*	The inappropriate sentence implies a gender binary bias.
She behaves like a woman as well as a man.	She is *gender fluid.* The person is gender fluid. She is *gender nonconforming.*	*Gender fluid* and *nonconforming* also avoid gender binary bias.
His *birth sex* was male.	His *sex assigned at birth* was male.	*Birth sex* minimizes the effects of sociocultural factors on gender identity.

B.2.2b. Use the Appropriate Terms of Gender Identities

Inappropriate	Write Correctly
Rachel is transgendered. We saw a transgender.	
He is a transvestite.	
Male-to-female transformed individual. Male-to-female transformed man.	
She is female-to-male transformed.	
He is a male-to-female transgender man.	
Our voice clinic serves only typical males and females.	
They are neither female nor male.	
Sometimes he behaves like a man and at other times like a woman.	*Hint:* Show variations
She was a girl according to her birth sex.	

B.2.3a. Use the Appropriate Terms of Sexual Orientations

- *Sexual orientation* (not *preference*) refers to sexual and emotional attraction one feels; terms include lesbian, gay men (but not *gays*), heterosexual (but not *homosexual*), straight, bisexual, queer, polysexual, pansexual, asexual, and other evolving terms.
- Write *sexual and gender minorities*, *sexual orientation and gender diversity*, or such abbreviations as *LGBTQIA+* (but not just *LGBT*) to refer to a group of persons with multiple gender identities and sexual orientations.

Incorrect	Correct	Note
Participants were 20 male and 20 female *homosexuals.*	Participants were 20 *gay men* and 20 *lesbians.*	Be specific as well as appropriate.
The language skills of 20 lesbians were compared with those of 20 *normal* women.	The language skills of 20 lesbians were compared with those of 20 *cisgender* women.	Avoid the implications of normality or abnormality.
Sexual orientation of the participants was not significant, although the *sex* of the participants was.	Sexual orientation of the participants was not significant, although the *gender* of the participants was.	The revised version avoids a potential confusion between gender and sexual orientation.
The family values of gay men were compared with *acceptable traditional* values.	The family values of gay men were compared with those of *heterosexual* (or *cisgender)* men.	The revision avoids the implication of *unacceptable* values of gay men.
The speech of lesbian mothers directed to their children was compared with those of the *standard* group.	The speech of lesbian mothers directed to their children was compared with the speech of *straight* (or *cisgender*) women.	The revision avoids the notion of standard set by one or the other group. Cisgender may replace *straight.*
We compared the voice characteristics of typical men with those of atypical men.	We compared the voice characteristics of *cisgender men* with those of a group of *gender minority.*	Though fine in other contexts, *typical* in this context may imply a bias of normality.

B.2.3b. Use the Appropriate Terms of Sexual Orientations

Incorrect	Write Correctly
Homosexual men and women were recruited for the study.	
Voice characteristics of 50 lesbians were compared with those of a group of *typical* women.	
Dysfluencies of men with *normal sexual orientation* were assessed along with those of gay men.	*Hint:* Use the term *heterosexual.*
A client's sex, not sexual orientation, may be a significant factor.	*Hint:* Use the term gender instead of sex.
The religious values of lesbians were compared with *acceptable traditional values.*	
We assessed the pragmatic language skills of a group of typical women with those of a group of atypical women.	

B.2.4a. Avoid Prejudicial Reference to Disabilities

- Describe disabilities objectively, avoiding sentimental, evaluative, or euphemistic terms.
- Generally, use the people-first language (not their disability); exceptionally, use the identity-first language, chosen by the members of a cultural group (e.g., the Deaf culture)
- Write Deaf with a capital *D* to describe persons with severe hearing loss who use a sign language.
- Do not use disabilities to suggest metaphoric meaning.

Incorrect	Correct	Note
The man was a *victim* of laryngeal cancer.	The man had laryngeal cancer.	Avoid such terms as *victim*, *suffers from*, *afflicted with*, and *crippled* because they suggest negative evaluations.
The child *suffers* from severe apraxia of speech.	The child's apraxia of speech is severe.	
The man with aphasia is *crippled*.	The man with aphasia has hemiplegia.	
The *stutterer* could not order in restaurants. The dysarthric woman's speech intelligibility was severely limited.	Mr. Jones, who stutters, could not order in restaurants. Ms. Smith's dysarthria severely limited her speech intelligibility.	The correct versions put the persons first, not their disabilities. *Dysarthric*, *aphasic*, and such other terms are adjectives, not nouns.
He has an extremely severe hearing disability.	He is a Deaf person.	For many, deafness is not a disability or a disorder.
Mr. Fine with paraplegia is *handi-capable*.	Mr. Fine with paraplegia is now able to stand without support.	Other euphemistic terms include *physically challenged* and *other-abled*.
The *wheelchaired* need access to our clinics.	People in wheelchairs need access to our clinic.	*Confined to wheelchair* is unacceptable, but *wheelchair user* is fine.
Supervisors are *blind* to our day-to-day problems.	Supervisors *do not appreciate* our day-to-day problems.	Metaphoric use of a disability.
We assessed 20 *brain-damaged* adolescents.	We assessed 20 adolescents with traumatic brain injury.	*Brain-damaged* is unacceptable; it is not a clinical diagnosis, either.

B.2.4b. Avoid Prejudicial Reference to Disabilities

Incorrect	Write Correctly
The child was a victim of bilateral clefts of the hard palate.	
The woman, afflicted with a laryngeal infection, has a voice disorder.	
Fifteen autistic children were recruited for the experimental group.	
The teachers' plea for more computers fell on deaf ears.	
This aphasic has lost her speech.	
The stutterer agreed to come for treatment.	
The dysarthric had prosodic problems.	
The wheelchair bound need easy access to buildings.	
We worked with 15 men with severe hearing impairment.	
Our sample consisted of 15 right-brain–damaged adult men.	

B.2.5a. Avoid Prejudicial Reference to Ethnic or Racial Identity

- Use the terms that ethnic or racial groups prefer to describe themselves.
- Use the more specific terms to general terms (e.g., the more specific *Chinese Americans* rather than the more general *Asian Americans*).
- Capitalize the racial and ethnic terms (e.g., *White* and *Black*, not *white* and *black*).

Incorrect	Correct	Note
Seven Afro-American children participated in the study.	Seven African American children participated in the study.	Do not hyphenate *African American*
The study included 25 *Hispanic* children.	The study included 25 Mexican American children.	Such terms as *Cuban American* or *Puerto Rican American* add specificity when needed.
Only a small number of *Native Americans* could be sampled.	Only a small number of Navajo Indians could be sampled.	*Native Americans* is fine, but specification (*Cherokee, Sioux*) is preferred.
A majority of subjects were *Orientals*.	A majority of subjects were Vietnamese.	*Oriental* is prejudicial; prefer the more specific term.
Our clients are mostly *Asians* living in New York City.	Our clients are mostly Asian Americans living in New York City. Our clients are mostly Chinese Americans living in New York City.	Asians live in Asia, and Asians living in the United States are *Asian Americans*. Prefer the specific group (e.g., *Thai American, Japanese American*).
We compared the speech sound productions of *White children* with those of *Black children*.	We compared the speech sound productions of White American children with those of Black American children.	White people are distributed globally; be specific (e.g., White European, White Canadian).
Indian Americans and *American Indians* refer to the same group of people.	Indian Americans and American Indians are different groups.	*Indian Americans* may be from India or may have Indian ancestry; *American Indians* are *Native Americans*.

B.2.5b. Avoid Prejudicial Reference to Ethnic or Racial Identity

Incorrect	Write Correctly
The prevalence of high blood pressure is high among Afro-American adults.	
We will select an equal number of white and black students for evaluation.	
Hispanic adults with a history of stroke will be recruited for the study.	
Native American participants did as well as any other ethnic group.	
The oriental clients did not exhibit the same characteristics as the White clients.	
We analyzed the literacy skills of White first graders and Asian American first graders.	
We analyzed the language skills of non-Whites of Alaska.	

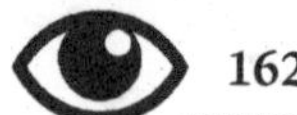

B.2.6a. Avoid Prejudicial Reference to Age

- Use appropriate terms for people of different ages (e.g., *child, adolescent, adult, older adult*)
- Consider the relevant gender identity of persons of any age that you describe (e.g., *gender-fluid girl, transgender boy, agender adolescent, male adolescent, transgender woman, cisgender man, genderqueer adult, etc.*; avoid *typical, atypical, normal,* and *abnormal*).
- Specify the ages, age ranges, the mean, and so forth; avoid such terms as *seniors, the aged, the elderly, older dependents, the senile,* and so forth; also avoid such nonspecific terms as *over 50, under 16,* and so forth.

Incorrect	Correct	Note
Our sample consisted of 50 *senior* citizens.	Our sample consisted of 50 individuals in the *age range of 65 to 75 years.*	*Senior* is both undesirable and nonspecific.
Most individuals with aphasia are *elderly.*	Most individuals with aphasia are *65 years and older.*	More specific age is specified.
Neurologically based communication disorders are more common in *the aged.*	Neurologically based communication disorders are more common among *older persons.*	*Older persons* is acceptable.
Old age is a *handicap* because of increased risk of dementia.	Incidence of dementia increases with *advancing age.*	Do not suggest that old age is a handicap.
The *aged* are more prone to *senility.*	*Older persons* have a higher risk of dementia.	*Dementia* is an accepted diagnostic term.
Last year, we served 200 girls of *atypical* gender identity.	Last year, we served 200 *agender a*dolescent girls aged *13 to 17 years* with a mean of 14 years.	Gender identity as well as the age range are specified.
The study sample included 15 women with normal sexual orientation in the age range of 25 to 35 (Mean = 30) and 15 transgender women in the same age range.	The study sample included 15 cisgender women in the age range of 25 to 35 years (mean = 30 years) and 15 transgender women in the same age range.	Correct gender identity, age range, and the mean are specified.

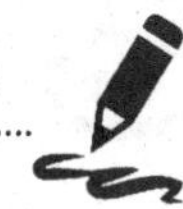

B.2.6b. Avoid Prejudicial Reference to Age

Incorrect	Correct
Our clients are mostly older dependents.	
Dysarthria is more common in the elderly than in the younger.	
Fifty percent of our annual caseload consists of persons over 50 years of age.	
Children under 15 respond better to treatment.	
Senior citizens are handicapped by their advancing age.	
We compared the vocal fundamental frequency of 20 normal women with that of 20 women whose gender identity was abnormal.	

B.2.7a. Avoid Prejudicial Comparisons of Study Groups

- Avoid *normal* versus *abnormal* comparisons
- Replace *normal* with *typically speaking, typically developing, children who did not have autism, adults without dysarthria*, and so forth.
- Replace *abnormal* with clinically specific diagnosis (*persons with aphasia, women with voice disorders, children who stutter*, and so forth).
- Use objective terms to describe such variables as socioeconomic status, income levels, education, those who receive government assistance, and so forth. See B.2. Terms for Writing Without Bias.

Incorrect	Correct	Note
We compared the dysfluency rates of children who stutter with those of *normal children.*	We compared the dysfluency rates of children who stutter with those of *children who were typically fluent.*	The revision avoids the implication that children who stutter are *abnormal.*
I recruited two groups of children: one with *acceptable language skills* and the other with *deviant* language.	I recruited two groups of children: one with *typically developing language* and the other with *speech sound disorders.*	*Typically developing* and *typically speaking* are acceptable alternatives. A diagnostic term should replace *deviant.*
The results of the *normal* and *clinical* group are presented in Table 1.	The results of Group 1 (*adults with typical speech*) and those of Group 2 (*persons with apraxia of speech*) are presented in Table 1.	*Clinical group* is an acceptable term, but specificity is better. *Experimental group* and *control group are acceptable alternatives.*
On a grammatical morphological test, children of *welfare mothers* scored 10% below the norm for their age.	On a grammatical morphological test, children of *mothers who received Temporary Assistance for Needy Families (TANF)* scored 10% below the norm for their age.	Avoid such terms as *welfare reliant, poverty stricken, poorly educated, homeless,* and so forth. See B.2. Terms for Writing Without Bias for acceptable alternatives.

B.2.7b. Avoid Prejudicial Comparisons of Study Groups

Incorrect	Write Correctly
We analyzed the turn-taking skills of normal children and those of children with specific language impairment.	
Dysfluency rates of regular children were lower than the rates of stuttering children.	*Hint:* Correct the two kinds of errors.
The adults in Group I had good speech, whereas those in Group 2 had poor speech.	*Hint:* Replace *good* and *poor*.
Children of poorly educated mothers may have limited pragmatic language skills.	*Hint:* Check B.2. Terms for Writing Without Bias for alternatives.
We examined the literacy resources available to children in low- and high- income families.	*Hint:* Specify income ranges.

B.3. Format of Scientific Writing

Margins

B.3.1. Leave Correct Margins

Margins should be 1 inch (2.54 cm) on the top, bottom, right, and left of every page. Use the specified margins on all papers you submit.

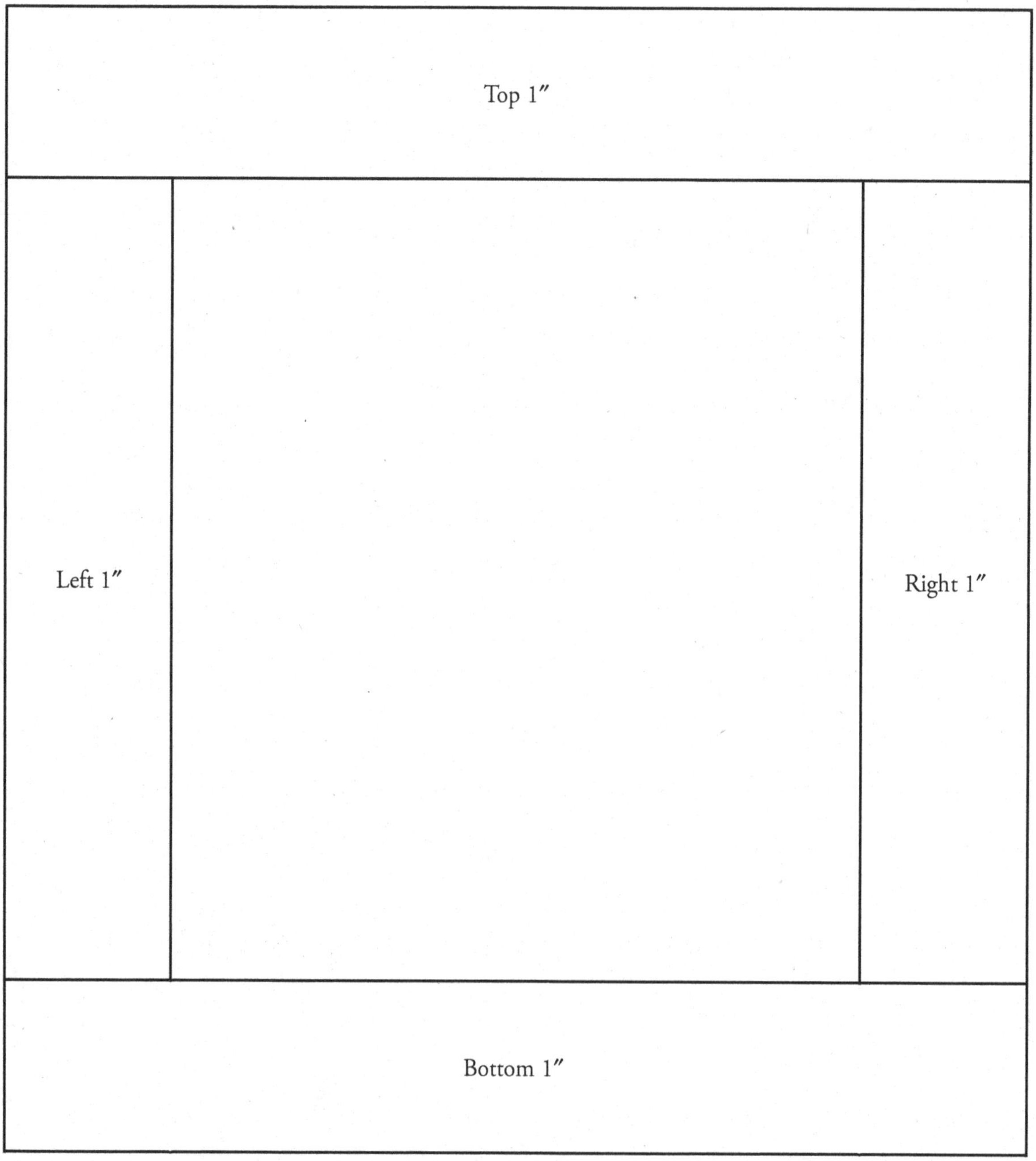

Title Page

B.3.2. Type Correctly the Title Page of a Paper for Publication

- Titles should be succinct.
- Limit the titles of journal articles to a maximum of 12 words.

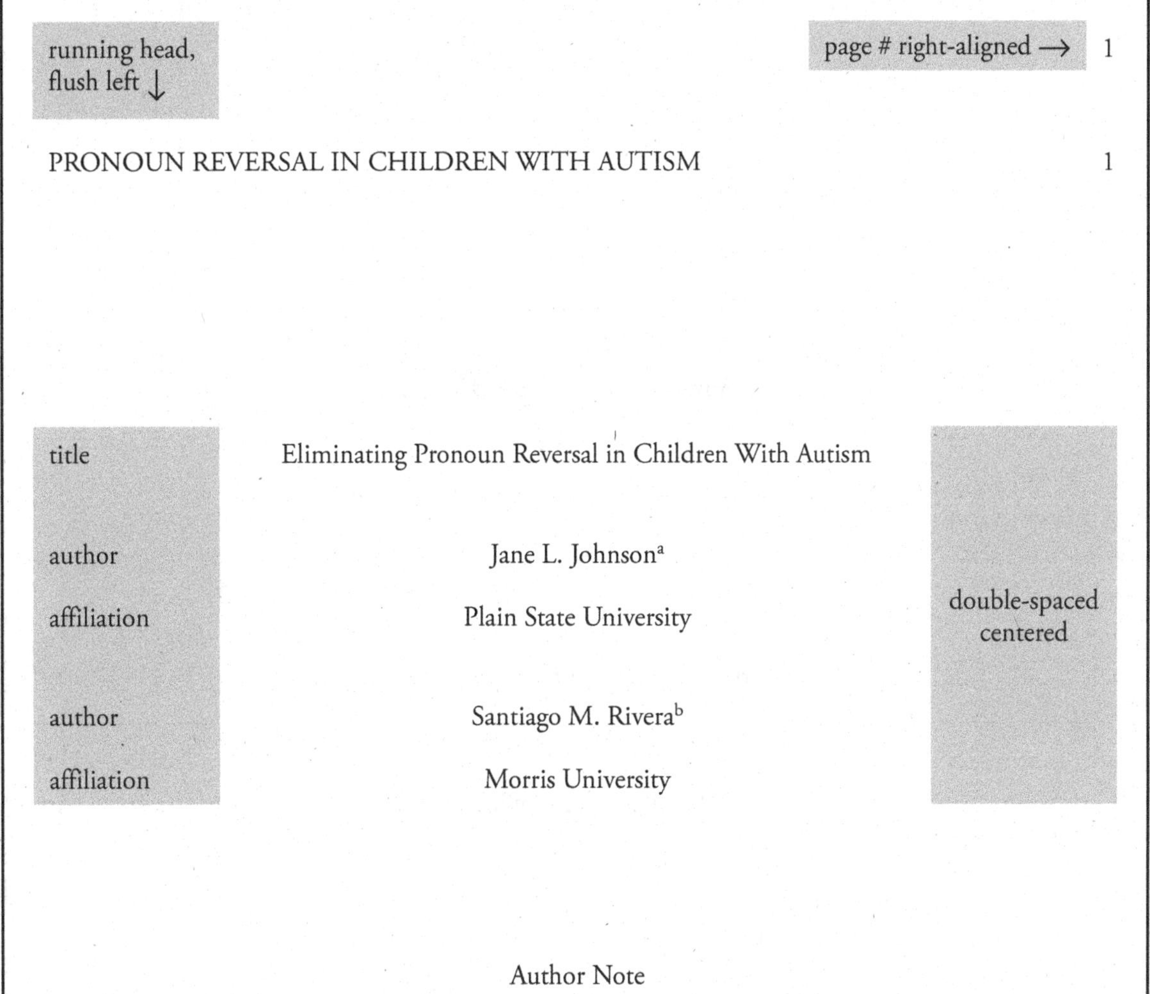

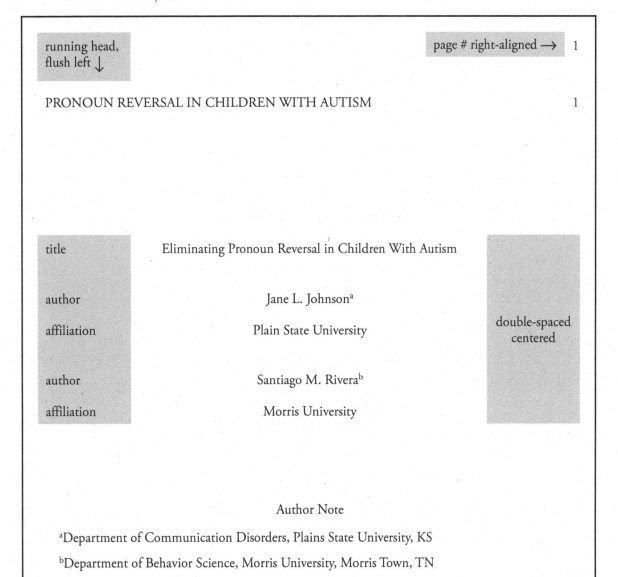

running head, flush left ↓

page # right-aligned ⟶ 1

PRONOUN REVERSAL IN CHILDREN WITH AUTISM 1

title: Eliminating Pronoun Reversal in Children With Autism

author: Jane L. Johnson[a]

affiliation: Plain State University

author: Santiago M. Rivera[b]

affiliation: Morris University

double-spaced centered

Author Note

[a]Department of Communication Disorders, Plains State University, KS

[b]Department of Behavior Science, Morris University, Morris Town, TN

We have no conflicts of interest to disclose.

Correspondence concerning this article should be addressed to Jane L. Johnson, Department of Communication Disorders, Plains State University, Plains, KS 03035. E-mail: jlj@plainstate.edu

Note: The author note also may contain acknowledgment of financial support, study registration, related reports, and change of author affiliation. See the *Publication Manual of the American Psychological Association* (7th ed., 2020; also referred to as APA Manual or APA style) for details.

B.3.3. Type Correctly the Title Page of a Class (Term) Paper

- All lines are double-spaced and centered.
- Type the paper due date.

page # right-aligned → 1

Recent Advances in Hearing Aid Technology

Toya Tinsley

Department of Speech-Language Pathology

Mountain State University

SLP 550 Aural Rehabilitation

Professor Melinda Malaisson Fall 2017

October 20, 2022

Running Head

B.3.4. Type the Manuscript Running Head Correctly

- Type a **running head**—a shorter version of the title of papers submitted for publication—at the top-left corner of **each page** (including the title page), except pages that contain figures.
- Insert the appropriate page number, right justified.
- The running head is printed on the right- or the left-hand page of published articles or books.
- Skip the running head on class papers submitted to instructors.

TREATING STUTTERING IN CHILDREN 1

Treating Stuttering in Children: A Review of Research

Indira M. Gonzalez[a]

Mountain State University

Author Note

[a]Department of Speech and Hearing Sciences, Mountain State University.

I have no known conflict of interest to disclose.

Correspondence concerning this article should be addressed to Indira M. Gonzalez, Department of Speech and Hearing Sciences. Mountain State University, Mountain, LS 76765. E-mail: indirag@mountainstate.edu

Abstract

B.3.5. Write an Abstract on the Second Page

- Type an abstract on the second page.
- Consult the journal to which the paper is to be submitted for the specific format.
- American Speech-Language-Hearing Association (ASHA) journals require a structured format: **Purpose, Method, Results, Conclusions** in bold; each section may contain a single paragraph; other journals may require a single paragraph without subheadings.
- Type the word **Abstract** at the top in bold font, centered on the page.
- Do not indent the first line of the paragraphs.
- Type the running head on the top-left corner and the page number on the top-right corner.
- Double-space the abstract.
- Do not exceed 250 words; however, check the guideline of the journal to which you plan to submit your paper; guidelines vary.
- Do not quote, but cite authors if necessary.
- Use abbreviations, but spell them out on their first use.
- Type all numbers as digits (except those that begin a sentence).
- See B.5.2 for more on *Abstracts.*

Abstract

Purpose: Pronoun reversal, a persistent language problem of children with autism spectrum disorder, has been difficult to eliminate. The purpose of this study was to test the possibility that echolalia, frequently found in children with autism, may contribute to pronoun reversal.

Method: Four children between 5 and 7 years of age, diagnosed with autism spectrum disorder, participated. Within a multiple baseline design across the four participants, I applied the time-out contingency on echolalia and measured the frequency of pronoun reversal.

Results: As the experimental contingency of time-out decreased the frequency of echolalia, the frequency of pronoun reversal was also decreased.

Conclusion: Echolalia is a likely contributor to pronoun reversal in children with autism spectrum disorder. Reducing echolalia with a time-out contingency may effectively reduce pronoun reversal.

Beginning of Text

B.3.6. Begin the Text With an Untitled Introductory Section on Page Three

- Type the title of the paper in bold font and center it. Do not type the author's name.
- Do not type Introduction as a heading.
- Indent each paragraph by 0.5 in.

PRONOUN REVERSAL IN CHILDREN WITH AUTISM 3

Eliminating Pronoun Reversal in Children With Autism

An Experimental Analysis

Among the many language characteristics of children with autism, echolalia and pronoun reversal occur frequently. **Echolalia** is the seemingly meaningless repetition of what is heard. **Pronoun reversal** refers to the substitution of an appropriate personal pronoun with an inappropriate pronoun. For example, a child with autism spectrum disorder may substitute *you* for *me,* and vice versa (Weathermeir, 2022).

[text continues]

Note: Defined terms may be italicized or printed in bold type. Also note that this boxed display does not show the required margins.

Heading Levels

B.3.7. Use the Headings Within the Text Consistently

- Make headings brief, direct, and relevant to the contents that follow.
- Use the word processor's *Style* menu to create easily repeatable headings.
- Organize an empirical report (with human participants or animal subjects) with standard headings of Method, Results, Discussion, References.
- Follow the instructor's guidelines to create headings and subheadings in an academic term paper.
- APA style includes up to five levels of heading; use the selected style consistently.
- Capitalize the first letter of only the major words of a heading and the first letter of all words that contain four letters or more (e.g., in a heading or title, the *a* in *and* will not be capitalized, but the *w* in *With* will be).
- Do not type *Introduction* at the beginning of a paper.
- Note that the *headings* appear within the text of an article, and the *title* is essentially the name of the article.
- Write more than one paragraph of text under a heading.
- Note that the journals of ASHA
  - use their own heading styles that differ from APA style
  - may not use a consistent heading style across its journals or within a single issue of a particular journal except for the standard headings (Method, Results, Discussion, Conclusion)
  - may use heading levels of different font sizes *and* font types (roman and italic) across its journals
  - follow the heading style of the particular ASHA journal to which the article is to be submitted.

Two Levels of Headings

Results

[Level 1; centered, boldfaced, upper- and lowercase heading.
The text begins with an indented paragraph on the next line.]

The results will be presented descriptively as well as statistically . . .

Treatment Effects

[Level 2; flush left, boldfaced, upper- and lowercase side heading; the text begins with an indented paragraph on the next line.]

Effects of the two treatments are presented in Figures 1 and 2 . . .

Three Levels of Headings

Method

[Level 1; centered, boldfaced, upper- and lowercase heading.]

Stimulus Selection

[Level 2; flush left, boldfaced, upper- and lowercase side heading; the text begins on the next line with an indented paragraph.]

We selected objects as well as colorful pictures for training stimuli . . .

Baseline Procedure. We established the baselines with 20 stimulus items . . .

[Level 3; indented, boldfaced, upper- and lowercase paragraph heading ending with a period. After one space, the text begins on the same line.]

Four Levels of Headings

Method

(Level 1; centered, boldfaced, upper- and lowercase heading.)

Assessment Materials

[Level 2; flush left, boldfaced, upper- and lowercase side heading. The text begins on the next indented line.]

We used both standardized assessment instruments and client-specific procedures prepared for each client . . .

Stimulus Pictures. We selected colorful pictures from various magazines . . .

[Level 3; indented, boldfaced, upper- and lowercase paragraph heading ending with a period. After one space, the text begins on the same line.]

Dependent Variables. We used several instruments to measure the dependent variables . . .

[Level 4; indented, boldfaced, italicized, upper- and lowercase paragraph heading ending with a period. After one space, the text begins on the same line.]

Five Levels of Heading

Experiment 1: Morphological Training

[Level 1; centered, boldfaced, upper- and lowercase heading.]

Participant Selection Procedure

[Level 2; flush left, boldfaced, upper- and lowercase heading; the text begins on the next indented line.]

We selected participants from the list of clients seeking services . . .

Stimulus Materials. We selected artist-drawn pictures to evoke the target responses . . .

[Level 3; indented, boldfaced, lowercase paragraph heading ending in a period. After one space, the text begins on the same line.]

Training Procedure. We used the discrete trial training procedure . . .

[Level 4; indented, boldfaced, italicized, lowercase paragraph heading ending in a period. After one space, the text begins on the same line.]

Probe Procedure. We used both the intermixed probe and pure probe methods . . .

[Level 5; Indented, italicized, upper- and lowercase paragraph heading ending in a period. After one space, the text begins on the same line.]

 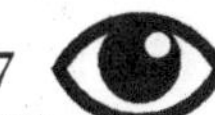

Note to Student Writers

The APA heading styles are required for research papers to be submitted to a journal that uses that style. Those heading styles also may be required for theses and dissertations. It is better to use the same style in term papers. Always using one style format, such as that of the APA, will make it easier to organize any kind of writing. Nonetheless, follow the guidelines provided by your instructor in each class and the journal to which you wish to submit your paper. As noted, the journals of ASHA generally use the APA style, but with some unique features.

Also, as noted in B.1. Introduction to Scientific Writing, books, including this one, do not fully conform to all aspects of the APA style. Books are uniquely designed to conform to the style of the publishing house and for aesthetic purposes. Therefore, APA style examples are not to be selected by looking at the stylistic aspects of this or any other book. As pointed out earlier, even some journals that purport to use the APA style may not adopt all aspects of it.

The actual style as seen in published papers of a particular journal may be a better guide.

Fonts and Font Size

B.3.8. Use Acceptable Fonts and Size

- *Serif* fonts have fine-line strokes that finish off the main strokes of letters (as the two small horizontal lines on **N**). *Sans serif* fonts lack the finer strokes (e.g., **N**). Both are acceptable.
- Select the font size depending on the font type, as noted next. Use them consistently throughout the paper.
- Type in the International Phonetic Symbols as needed. They are available online.

Font Type and Size	Unacceptable	Note
Serif Times New Roman, 12-point; Georgia, 11-point Sans Serifs Calibri and Arial 11-point; Lucida 10-point Use a sans serif for labels and legends within figures (between 8 and 14 points). 10-point for footnotes	Exotic and ornamental fonts Cursive fonts Condensed fonts Very large or very small sizes	Check the recommended font type and size for the journal to which you submit.

B.3.9. Use Bold Font Correctly

- Journal articles generally do not bold words within the text.
- In term papers and other kinds of writing, use bold if permitted.
- See B.4.9 and B.4.10 for correct italicizing.

Use Bold For	Examples	Note
Terms when they are defined	**Semantics** is the study of meaning.	Do not use bold for subsequent use of the term.
L1 through L4 headings *y*- and *x*-axis titles in graphs Table Number Figure number	**Bilingualism** (Level 1) **Sequential Bilingualism** (Level 2) **Percent Correct** (*y*) **Session Number** (*x*) **Table 1.** **Figure 5.**	Do not bold the table or figure titles.

Page Numbers

B.3.10. Number the Pages Correctly

Do	Do Not	Note
Place the page number on the top-right corner, five spaces to the right of the running head.	Give a new identity to the inserted pages (e.g., 32A, 59B).	Use the *Header* command of the word processor to automatically insert page numbers and the running heads. Format page numbers as a right-aligned paragraph to print them at the end of the right margin.
Number all pages of the paper consecutively, including the title page, reference list, tables, appendixes, and other end materials.		
Renumber or repaginate the entire paper when you delete or add pages.		

B.3.11. Reprint the Corrected Pages

Do	Do Not	Note
Reprint or retype the corrected pages.	Use handwritten corrections on your paper.	Final submission should be free from distracting corrections.

Line Spacing and Line Length

B.3.12. Use Appropriate Line Spacing

Double Space	Triple Space	Single Space
title page entire paper all headings all text quotations tables (single spacing is acceptable) figure legends reference lists initial drafts of clinical reports	Before starting a major heading (optional). Before displayed equations.	Single space no portion of a research or term paper, except for the table entries, which may be single, 1.5, or double spaced. Footnotes in a research paper are single spaced. **Exception:** The final versions of clinical reports and all forms of correspondence. These are always single spaced.

B.3.13. Align the Text to the Left Margin

Left Alignment	Do Not	Note
Use the flush-left style. Do not break words at the end of a line by using a hyphen.	Right- or full-justify the lines; let them look ragged at the right margin.	Justified text will have uneven spaces between words, but the line length will be equal.

B.3.14. Correct the Spelling Errors

Do	Do Not	Note
Keep the word processor's spellchecker turned on to make online corrections. Manually double-check the spelling yourself, preferably on printed pages.	Depend entirely on the word processor's spellchecker. Depend entirely on the spellchecker's autocorrection feature.	If you typed *he* for *the*, the spellchecker will not highlight it because *he* is a word in the dictionary. The autocorrection feature may insert a wrong word.

B.4. Elements of Scientific Style

Capitalization

B.4.1. Capitalize the First Words

Capitalize	Examples	Note
The first letter of the first word in a sentence	This does not concern you.	
The first letter of the first word after a colon that begins a complete sentence	One thing is certain: No one has made a perfect study.	
The first letter of the first word and the first letter of the first word after a colon when referencing a book or an article in the reference list	Bowen, J. (1998). *Joy of journalism: One woman's journey*. Premier Press. Tan, K. (2001). Ecstasy of scientific writing: A tutorial. *Journal of Scientific Writing, 55,* 23–45.	Italicize the book titles, journal titles, and journal volume numbers.

B.4.2. Capitalize the First and the Major Words

Capitalize	Examples	Note
Book and article titles specified in the text	Although the article, "Neuroscience: A Tutorial" is good, the book *Neuroscience of Communication* is more comprehensive.	The article title is enclosed within quotation marks; the book title is italicized. In the *References* list, capitalize only the first word of a book title and the first word after a colon.
Names of specific university departments	Department of English, California State University–Fresno	A *department of English* (unspecified)
Titles of specific university courses	CSD 200 Introduction to Research Methods	A *course on research methods* (unspecified)
Specific test titles	Test of Early Language Development	A *test on language development* (unspecified)

B.4.3. Capitalize the Words Correctly in Headings

<table>
<tr><th>Capitalize</th><th>Examples</th><th>Note</th></tr>
<tr><td>Major words in heading levels 1 and 2, including grammatical words with four or more letters</td><td>Method
(L1)
Dependent Variables
(L2)
Persons With Aphasia
(L2)</td><td rowspan="2">Do not capitalize the conjunction and as well as articles a and the in the headings.
See the section, B.3.7. Use the Headings Within the Text Consistently.
No heading style has all capital letters.</td></tr>
<tr><td>only the first word in level 3, 4, and 5 (indented paragraph) headings in which the text begins after the heading</td><td>Baseline procedures. (L3)
Probe procedures. (L4)
Group A Results. (L5)</td></tr>
</table>

B.4.4. Capitalize Proper Nouns and Trade Names

Capitalize	Examples	Note
All proper nouns and trade names in the text, the headings, and the reference list	Skinnerian conditioning Pavlovian experiments The Lombard effect Microsoft Word Adobe Acrobat	Note that in the first two examples, the second word is not capitalized. Do not capitalize *eustachian tube* and *cesarean section* unless they start a sentence.

B.4.5. Capitalize the Chapters and Sections the Reader Is Referred To

Capitalize	Examples	Note
Section titles or book chapters in the same article or book the reader is referred to	As pointed out in the Discussion section . . . See Chapter 4 for details.	However: *The discussion section in a paper . . .* *Several chapters of a book . . .*

 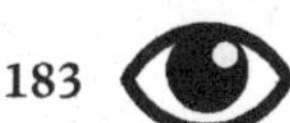

B.4.6. Capitalize Nouns That Are Followed by a Number or Letter

Capitalize	Examples	Note
Nouns followed by a numeral or a letter	As shown in Table 7 . . . As described in Document QZ As specified in Section 9(b) During Trial 9	However, *the article did not contain any tables, documents, sections, and trials . . .*

B.4.7. Capitalize Both Words in Otherwise Capitalized Hyphenated Compound

Capitalize	Examples	Note
The first letter of both words in the case of a hyphenated compound word that needs to be capitalized	The HIV-AIDS risk factors . . . The client is of Anglo-Irish background.	The rule applies only if the term is otherwise capitalized; see B.4.8. for exceptions.

B.4.8. Do Not Capitalize the Second Word of a Hyphenated Compound in Reference Lists

Do Not Capitalize	Examples	Note
The first letter of the second word of a hyphenated compound word in reference lists	Barr, B. (2022). Long-term effects of stuttering therapy. *Journal of Stuttering Therapy, 55*, 28–38. Kang, U. (2019). *Accident-prone adults and traumatic brain injury*. Thomson.	The rule applies to entries in a reference list; see also, B4.7. However, *HIV-AIDS* in the reference list as well (words that are always capitalized)

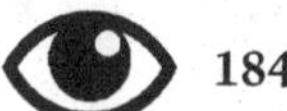

Italicization

B.4.9. Use Italics Correctly Within the Body of Text

- Underline if you cannot italicize (as in handwriting and typing on an old typewriter).

<table>
<tr><th>Use Italics For</th><th>Examples</th><th>Note</th></tr>
<tr><td>Specific book or journal titles in text citations</td><td>Allport's classic book, Introduction to Psychology, is excellent.

An ASHA journal, American Journal of Audiology</td><td rowspan="2">Capitalize all major words of book titles in the text, but only the first letter of the first word in the reference list.

Capitalize all major words of journals in the text and the reference list.

See B.4.10.</td></tr>
<tr><td>Names of journals</td><td>The Journal of Mind, is good for the mentalists.</td></tr>
<tr><td>An undefined new, technical, or key term when first introduced</td><td>The term phonology does not refer to a skill.

Cognition is a surrogate for observable behaviors.</td><td rowspan="5">Do not italicize the following:

a posteriori

a priori

et al.

per se</td></tr>
<tr><td>Terms or morphemes that denote linguistic examples</td><td>I taught the present progressive ing and the pronouns he and she.

The plural morpheme s cannot stand alone.</td></tr>
<tr><td>Letters used as statistical symbols or algebraic variables</td><td>t test

trial c</td></tr>
<tr><td>Category names in a rating scale</td><td>A rating of 1 means excellent

and 2 means good.</td></tr>
</table>

B.4.10. Use Reverse Italics Correctly

Reverse italics means the same as the roman font.

Use Reverse Italics For	Examples	Note
Another book title within a book title that is italicized.	In the text: Perkins (2010), in his book *Fantastic Speech Motor Theories: Johnson's* Modules of Motor Control, criticized Johnson for proposing a speculative model.	In the reference list: Perkins, K. (2010). *Fantastic Speech Motor Theories: Johnson's* Modules of Motor Control. Modular Press. Note that Perkins's book title contains another book title. The book title within a title is in roman font.

B.4.11. Use Italics Correctly in the Reference List

Use Italics For	Examples	Note
Book titles	*Introduction to communicative disorders*	Capitalize only the first word.
Names of journals and their volume numbers	*Journal of Human Communication, 52*	Capitalize all major words.
Titles of unpublished papers presented at conventions, meetings, and symposia	Crosslin, J. (2020, April). *Noun phrase training.* Paper presented at the Tennessee Conference on Language Disorders, Memphis, TN.	See the section, Reference List.

Hyphenation

B.4.12. Use the Hyphen Correctly

- Follow the guidelines given in *Merriam-Webster's Dictionary* or the unabridged edition of *Webster's* dictionary (the APA *Manual*'s recommendation).
- Check the current usage because many hyphenated words eventually lose the hyphen.

Incorrect	Correct	Note
Schedule follow up assessments.	Schedule follow-up assessments.	*Follow-up* as a noun (or adjective) is hyphenated. *Follow up* as a verb is not hyphenated.
role playing method	role-playing method	Hyphenate a compound with a participle when it precedes the term it modifies.
anxiety arousing situations	anxiety-arousing situations	
food deprived animals	food-deprived animals	
trial by trial analysis	trial-by-trial analysis	Hyphenate an adjectival phrase when it precedes the term it modifies.
minute by minute scoring	minute-by-minute scoring	
to be probed stimuli	to-be-probed stimuli	
high achievement group	high-achievement group	Hyphenate an adjective-and-noun compound when it precedes the term it modifies.
middle class families	middle-class families	
low frequency sounds	low-frequency sounds	
six item test	six-item test	Hyphenate a compound that begins with a number and the compound that precedes the term it modifies.
two way analysis of variance	two-way analysis of variance	
5 s duration	5-s duration	
fifth grade children	fifth-grade children	
pro Freudian	pro-Freudian	Compounds in which the base word is capitalized
post Skinnerian	post-Skinnerian	
pre 1990 post 2000	pre-1990 post-2000	Compounds in which the base word is a number
post COVID pre ASHA	post-COVID pre-ASHA	Compounds in which the base word is an abbreviation

Use the hyphen correctly *(continued)*

Incorrect	Correct	Note
recount (*count again*)	re-count (not *recount*)	Words that could be mistaken without a hyphen
recover (*cover again*)	re-cover (not *recover*)	
recreate (*create again*)	re-create (not *recreation*)	
resend (send again)	re-send (not *resend*)	
self concept	self-concept	All *self-* compounds used as nouns or adjectives
self scored quiz	self-scored quiz	
self examination	self-examination	
metaanalysis	meta-analysis	Hyphen separates the same vowel or consonant in the compound word. *Exception*: prefixes *re* and *pre*; see B4.13.
antiintellectual	anti-intellectual	
cooccurrence	co-occurrence	
	sword-dance	
client centered counseling	client-centered counseling (*However*, The counseling was client centered.)	Use the hyphen when a compound adjective precedes the word it modifies. Do not use the hyphen when the compound adjective follows the word it modifies, as shown in parenthetical examples.
same sex children	same-sex children (*However*, The children were of the same sex.)	
user friendly program	user-friendly program (*However*, The program was user friendly.)	
student oriented exam	student-oriented exam (*However*, The exam was student oriented.)	
the low, moderate, and high anxiety groups	the low-, moderate-, and high-anxiety groups	When the base word (*anxiety* in the first example) is used only with the last modifier in a series of compound modifiers (*low*, *moderate*, and *high* in the same example), use the hyphen as shown.
5 and 10 sec time-out durations	5- and 10-sec time-out durations	
teacher and student centered	teacher- and student-centered	
long and short term treatment	long- and short-term treatment	

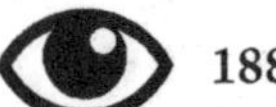

B.4.13. Do Not Overuse or Misuse the Hyphen

- Note, however, usage varies. Certain terms that start out as separate or hyphenated words eventually become solid words; consult *Webster's* for correct usage.

Incorrect	Correct	Note
health-care programs	health care programs	Do not use hyphens if the term is well established and the meaning is clear without it.
dysfluency-rates	dysfluency rates	
sex-role differences	sex role differences	
rank-order correlation	rank order correlation	
life-style changes	lifestyle changes	
data-base	database	
neurologically-based	neurologically based	Do not hyphenate words that end in *ly* and the ones that follow.
bi-lingual child	bilingual child	These prefixes are not followed by a hyphen. See *Webster's* for additional examples. However, *meta-analysis*
co-operate	cooperate	
counter-balanced design	counterbalanced design	
extra-sensory	extrasensory	
infra-structure	infrastructure	
inter-dental	interdental	
intra-observer reliability	intraobserver reliability	
macro-cephaly	macrocephaly	
mega-byte	megabyte	
meta-cognition	metacognition	
micro-computer	microcomputer	
mid-section	midsection	
mini-series	miniseries	See *Webster's* for many more examples.
multi-lingual	multilingual	
non-clinical	nonclinical However, non-Christian, non-Chinese	*Exception*: All capitalized nouns preceded by *non-*
over-qualified	overqualified	
post-test	posttest	
post-test	posttest	

Do not overuse or misuse the hyphen (*continued*)

Incorrect	Correct	Note
pre-test	pretest	
pre-experimental	preexperimental	Exceptions to the rule of hyphenating two words that end and begin with the same vowel (e-e).
re-engineer	reengineer	
re-evaluate re-examine	reevaluate reexamine	
pro-revolutionary pro-war	prorevolutionary prowar	However, *pro-Darwinian*
pseudo-science pseudo-logic	pseudoscience pseudologic	See *Webster* for many such examples
semi-annual semi-literate	semiannual semiliterate	
socio-economic psycho-linguistics	socioeconomic psycholinguistics	
sub-test sub-division	subtest subdivision	
super-script super-ordinate	superscript superordinate	
supra-glottal supra-orbital	supraglottal supraorbital	
ultra-sensitive ultra-liberal	ultrasensitive ultraliberal	
un-conditioned un-defined	unconditioned undefined	
under-funded over-emphasize	underfunded overemphasize	
web-site web-page	website webpage	
e-book e-reader	ebook ereader	
log-in	log in (verb)	Login page (noun)

Indentation

B.4.14. Use Correct Indentation

Indent	Do Not Indent	Note
0.5 in.: The first line of each paragraph of the text Level 4 and 5 paragraph style headings The second and subsequent paragraphs of block quotations	Abstracts Article titles Flush left Heading 2 and 3 Titles of tables and notes Legends of figure captions The first paragraph of block quotations The first line of each reference entry	Level 1 headings and titles are **centered**. Unindented lines are *flush left*. To indent paragraphs uniformly, use the word processor's default setting (typically five spaces), set your own tab settings, or format the paragraphs in *style* feature of the word processor.

Space After Punctuation

B.4.15. Give Correct Space or No Space After Punctuation

Correct	Number of Spaces
	One space after
Her data were valid. But no one cared. He said, "Let's go!" She asked, "Go where?"	A period and other punctuation marks at the end of sentences (e.g., !, ?)
Speech, language, and hearing	Commas
The clinician said: "Stop!"	Colons
These rules are vague; but follow them!	Semicolons
Penn, P. Z. (1993). Q. X. Zenkin	Each period that separates initials in names
	One space between
Penn, P. Z. (1999). *Nation of children.* Infancy Press.	Each element in a reference list
	One space on either side of
10 – 5 is 5. (minus sign)	A minus sign preceded and followed by a number
	One space before, but no space after
The negative value was –70.	A minus sign followed by a number
	No space after
p.m.; i.e.; U.S.	Internal periods in abbreviations
The ratio is 4:1.	Around colons in ratios
	No space before or after
The yet-to-be published book The client—a professional singer—came to the clinic with a hoarse voice. (dashes) (two typed hyphens with no space on either side become—.)	Single hyphens Double hyphens (*em dash*) Most word processors automatically convert two typed hyphens into one long hyphen (em dash) if no space is placed on either side of the hyphens.
I completed my studies during the 2016–2017 academic year.	An *en dash* is longer than a hyphen but shorter than an em dash. Select an en dash from the Insert Symbol menu.

Abbreviations

B.4.16a. Write Out Abbreviations the First Time You Use the Term, and Enclose the Abbreviations in Parentheses

- Do not write out abbreviations that are (a) defined as words in dictionaries (IQ, AIDA); (b) Latin (e.g., viz.); (c) time (hr, min); (d) measurement (cm, ml); and (e) statistical (SD, *t*, *p*).
- Abbreviate only to save space while retaining clarity of writing; do not abbreviate if it is to be used only a few times (three times or less).
- Spell it out if too many similar-sounding abbreviations clutter the writing and confuse the reader.
- Once selected, use the abbreviation consistently.

First Correct Citation	Subsequent Correct Citation	Note
The hearing threshold level (HTL) was measured . . .	The HTL was . . .	These audiological abbreviations need not be spelled out even the first time if an audiogram that spells them out accompanies the report.
A value of 100 hertz (Hz) means that . . .	I presented a tone of 200 Hz.	
A decibel (dB) is one tenth of a bel.	In 5-dB increments . . .	
The anatomy of the temporo-mandibular joint (TMJ) . . .	The TMJ is important for . . .	
We measured the mean length of utterance (MLU) in syllables.	The obtained MLU values are shown in Table 1.	
We presented a conditioned stimulus (CS).	We increased the intensity of the CS.	
You must obtain your Certificate of Clinical Competence (CCC).	Those who hold their CCC may practice independently.	Periods are not added to capitalized abbreviations.
Our professional organization is the American Speech-Language-Hearing Association (ASHA).	The president of ASHA spoke at the convention.	

B.4.17a. Do Not Start a Sentence With a Lowercase Abbreviation

Incorrect	Correct	Note
dB is one tenth of a bel.	The dB is one tenth of a bel.	The correct examples show the subsequent citations of the abbreviated words, which were spelled out earlier.
ppb* is useful in measuring the amount of pesticides in water.	The amount of the residual pesticide in water is measured in ppb.	
m, being a measure of micrometer . . .	Being a measure of micrometer, m is . . .	
ns is a very brief time period.	I used a special equipment to measure the ns.	

*ppb: parts per billion; ns: nanosecond.

Abbreviations

B.4.16b. Write Out Abbreviations the First Time You Use the Term and Enclose the Abbreviations in Parentheses

Incorrect First Citation	Rewrite Correctly
The ASHA *Code of Ethics* is an important document. The members of the American Speech-Language-Hearing Association should adhere to the code.	
In hearing evaluation, the SDT should be obtained. The speech detection threshold is the hearing level at which a person is just aware of speech.	
A loud noise is a UCS for startle response. The presentation of an unconditioned stimulus results in an unconditioned response.	
The LAD is essential for language learning. Without the language acquisition device, the child would be lost in confusion.	
In DRO, you specify the behavior that will not be reinforced. The effectiveness of the differential reinforcement of other behavior is well established.	
The child has a PE tube. Surgically implanted pressure-equalizing tubes allow for middle ear ventilation.	

B.4.17b. Do Not Start a Sentence With a Lowercase Abbreviation

Incorrect	Write Correctly
cc, being a metric measure . . .	
lb is a popular measure in the United States.	
min is an abbreviation for minutes.	
ms is longer than ns.	

cc: cubic centimeter; lb: pound; ms: millisecond.

B.4.18a. Use Latin Abbreviations Only in Parenthetical Constructions

- In nonparenthetical sentences, write their English equivalents; do not use Latin abbreviations in conversational speech.

Abbreviation	English Equivalent
etc.	and so forth
e.g.,	for example
i.e.,	that is
viz.,	namely
cf.	compare
vs.	versus, against

Exceptions:

1. Use the abbreviation v. for versus when referring to court cases: The historic *Brown v. Board of Education* ruling.
2. Use the Latin abbreviation et al. ("and others") in roman font in both the parenthetical and nonparenthetical constructions. See B.4.31. and B.4.32. for examples.

Incorrect	Correct
Pictures, objects, line drawings, etc., will be used as stimuli.	Pictures, objects, line drawings, and so forth, will be used as stimuli. A variety of stimuli (pictures, objects, line drawings, etc.) will be used.
Various reinforcers, e.g., tokens, stickers, and points, will be used as reinforcers.	Various reinforcers, for example, tokens, stickers, and points, will be used as reinforcers. Various reinforcers (e.g., tokens, stickers, and points) will be used.
The continuous reinforcement schedule, i.e., the fixed ratio 1 (FR1), may be used.	The continuous reinforcement schedule, that is, the fixed ratio 1 (FR1), may be used. The basic reinforcement schedule (i.e., the fixed ratio 1) may be used.
Certain variables, viz., the severity of the disorder and treatment intensity may influence the treatment outcome.	Certain variables, namely, the severity of the disorder and treatment intensity, may influence the treatment outcome. Certain variables (viz., the severity of the disorder and treatment intensity) may influence the treatment outcome.
Nativism vs. empiricism is a historical topic of discussion.	Nativism versus empiricism is a historical topic of discussion. The two opposing views (nativism vs. empiricism) are a historical topic of discussion.

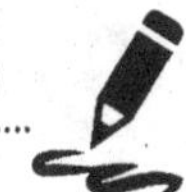

B.4.18b. Use Latin Abbreviations Only in Parenthetical Constructions

- Take note of an exception, however. Write both the forms of correct sentences except for the last.

Incorrect	Write Correctly
The various types of dysfluency including interjections, prolongations, repetitions, etc. characterize stuttered speech.	
Newer types of hearing aids, e.g., the digital aids, can reduce background noise.	
Neural hearing loss, i.e., the type of loss with nerve damage, may be severe.	
Many variables, viz., heredity, environmental toxicity, and maternal alcoholism can cause intellectual disability.	
Behaviorism vs. cognitivism is a good topic for debate.	
The Brown versus the Board of Education ruling forced racial integration in public schools.	

B.4.19a. Add the Lowercase Plural Morpheme *s* to Plural Abbreviations Without an Apostrophe

Incorrect	Correct	Note
ABR's, ECG's, EEG's, IQ's, Ed's., vol's.	ABRs, ECGs, EEGs, IQs, Eds. (for *Editors*), vols. (for volumes)	A common mistake is to add an apostrophe.

B.4.20a. With Abbreviations, Use the Period Correctly

Add Periods To	Do Not Add Periods To
Initials of names (Z. Q. Xompompin)	Degree abbreviations: AuD, PhD, EdD, MD, DDS, JD, MA, MS, RN, MSW, BA, BS, and others
Geographic names (U.S. Military)	
U.S. as an adjective (U.S. Department of Health and Human Services)	Capital letter abbreviations and acronyms: ASHA, APA, UNESCO, IQ
Latin abbreviations: *i.e., cf., vs., a.m., e.g.,*	Abbreviations of state names: CA, ND
Reference abbreviations: *Vol. 5,* 2nd ed., p. 10, paras. 5–9, Supp.	Measurement abbreviations: cm (centimeter), ml (milliliter), hr (hour), min (minute), s (seconds), kg (kilogram), ft (foot), lb (pound)
In era specifications: B.C.E., C.E., B.C., A.D.	*Exception:* Add a period to in. (inch) as it could be misread without the period.

B.4.21a. Abbreviate Units of Measurement When a Number Is Specified

Incorrect	Correct	Note
20 seconds 2 hours 20 kilograms 5 centimeters 29 percent	20 s 2 hr 20 kg 5 cm 29%	In scientific papers, units of time and other measures are abbreviated and always singular (e.g., kg, *not* kgs). Unless they are at the end of a sentence, there is no period at the end of these abbreviations. *Exception: in.* (for inch; a period is always added).

Note: In the noun phrase, no hyphen is used between the number and the abbreviation (20 s); a hyphen is used in an adjectival phrase (as in *a 20-s interval will be used*).

B.4.19b. Add the Lowercase Plural Morpheme *s* to Plural Abbreviations Without an Apostrophe

Incorrect	Write Correctly
HTL's	
MLU's	
SRT's	
FR's (for Fixed Ratio of Reinforcement)	

B.4.20b. With Abbreviations, Use the Period Correctly

Incorrect	Write Correctly
US Park Service	
Secretary, US Department of Labor	
viz	
etc	
Au.D.	

B.4.21b. Abbreviate Units of Measurement When a Number Is Specified

Incorrect	Write Correctly
10 minutes	
10 feet	
5 pounds	
5 seconds	
15 centimeters	
2 hours	

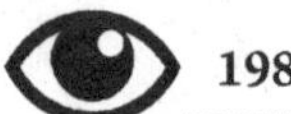

Numbers in Words or Numerals

B.4.22a. Write Out Units of Measurement When a Number Is Not Specified

Incorrect	Correct	Note
The weight was specified in kg. The specified weight was 10 kilograms.	The weight was specified in kilograms. The specified weight was 10 kg.	A specified number is always followed by an abbreviated unit of measure. An unspecified unit of measure is always followed by a word, not an abbreviation.
measured in cm . . . It was 10 centimeters long.	measured in centimeters . . . It was 10 cm long.	
several lb of sugar . . . You have 10 pounds of sugar.	several pounds of sugar . . . You have 10 lb of sugar.	
calculated the % of dysfluencies . . . The client had a 10 percent dysfluency rate.	calculated the percentage of dysfluencies . . . The client had a 10% dysfluency rate.	

B.4.23a. Use Roman Numerals Only When It Is an Established Practice

Incorrect	Correct
Cranial nerve 4	Cranial nerve IV
Type 2 error	Type II error
King George 3rd	King George III

B.4.24a. Use Arabic Numerals for Numbers 10 and Above

- However, see exceptions under B.4.25.

Incorrect	Correct	Note
I selected eleven participants.	I selected 11 participants.	Numbers 10 and above are not written in words unless they start a sentence.
The client is seventy-five years old.	The client is 75 years old.	
The client met the training criterion on the fifteenth trial.	The client met the training criterion on the 15th trial.	
The client's dysfluency was twenty percent.	The client's dysfluency was 20%.	

Numbers in Words or Numerals

B.4.22b. Write Out Units of Measurement When a Number Is Not Specified

Incorrect	Write Correctly
You can take several mg without side effects.	
The voice onset time of persons who stutter was slower by several ms.	
This task may take many hr.	

- mg: milligrams; ms: milliseconds.

B.4.23b. Use Roman Numerals Only When It Is an Established Practice

Incorrect	Write Correctly
Cranial nerve 8	
Type one error	
Pope Paul the 6th	

B.4.24b. Use Arabic Numerals for Numbers 10 and Above

Incorrect	Write Correctly
A caseload of fifty-five is large.	
The client met the training criterion in only twelve trials.	
The client's baserate production was fifteen percent.	
There are ten clients on the waiting list.	
She is twenty five years old.	

B.4.25a. Use Numerals for Numbers Below 10 in Specified Contexts

Generally, numerals below 10 are written out in words. There are exceptions, however. Numbers below 10 are written in numerals when they

- are grouped for comparison with numbers 10 or above
- precede a unit of measurement
- represent statistical or mathematical functions
- represent time, dates, ages, sample, number of participants in a study, scores on a scale, exact amounts of money, and items in a quantitative series

<table>
<tr><th>Incorrect</th><th>Correct</th><th>Note</th></tr>
<tr><td>I answered only nine out of 12 questions.</td><td>I answered only 9 out of 12 questions.</td><td rowspan="6">In each of these examples, a number below 10 is compared with a number 10 or above.
Therefore, even the numbers below 10 are written in numerals.</td></tr>
<tr><td>Stimuli include five pictures, three toys, and 12 objects.</td><td>Stimuli include 5 pictures, 3 toys, and 12 objects.</td></tr>
<tr><td>The ninth graders did better than the 12th graders.</td><td>The 9th graders did better than the 12th graders.</td></tr>
<tr><td>The fourth and 15th participants did not do well.</td><td>The 4th and the 15th participants did not do well.</td></tr>
<tr><td>Of the 15 clients, four dropped out of therapy.</td><td>Of the 15 clients, 4 dropped out of therapy.</td></tr>
<tr><td>Only seven of the 20 probe responses were correct.</td><td>Only 7 of the 20 probe responses were correct.</td></tr>
<tr><td>I used three lb of sugar.</td><td>I used 3 lb of sugar.</td><td rowspan="2">Numbers precede units of measurement.</td></tr>
<tr><td>I took a five-mg tablet.</td><td>I took a 5-mg tablet.</td></tr>
<tr><td>I divided it by seven.</td><td>I divided it by 7.</td><td rowspan="3">Numbers with statistical or mathematical functions.</td></tr>
<tr><td>A dysfluency rate of five % is high.</td><td>A dysfluency rate of 5% is high.</td></tr>
<tr><td>The third quartile.</td><td>The 3rd quartile.</td></tr>
<tr><td>The experiment took two weeks.</td><td>The experiment took 2 weeks.</td><td rowspan="6">Numbers that represent time, date, age, and so forth. Number in a series (of tables and pages, in this case).</td></tr>
<tr><td>I completed the degree in four years.</td><td>I completed the degree in 4 years.</td></tr>
<tr><td>The participants were four-year olds.</td><td>The subjects were 4-year-olds.</td></tr>
<tr><td>She scored six on a 7-point scale.</td><td>She scored 6 on a 7-point scale.</td></tr>
<tr><td>Please see Table Five.</td><td>Please see Table 5.</td></tr>
<tr><td>You can find this on page seven.</td><td>You can find this on page 7.</td></tr>
</table>

B.4.25b. Use Numerals for Numbers Below 10 in Specified Contexts

Incorrect	Write Correctly
I scored only six out of 12 answers.	
The seventh graders did better than the 11th graders.	
The third and 12th participants did not do well.	
Of the 17 clients, six needed booster treatment.	
The client's responses were correct on the seventh and 11th trials.	
I bought five kg of pesticide.	
The normal dosage is three mg.	
Multiply this number by four.	
An error rate of seven % is unacceptable.	
I completed the study in four weeks.	
I had seven-year-olds as participants.	
He scored five on a 7-point scale.	
Please see page nine.	
These data are presented in Figure four.	
Find the details in Chapter two.	

B.4.26a. Write Out in Words Numbers Below 10 in Specified Contexts

Take note of exceptions to this rule in B.4.25. Use words instead of numerals to write numbers that are

- not precisely measured values
- not set in comparison with numbers 10 and above
- the numbers zero and one in most (but not all) cases
- common fractions
- traditionally expressed only in words

Incorrect	Correct	Note
Such instances are few; perhaps 3 or 4.	Such instances are few; perhaps three or four.	Precise measurement is not implied.
The client repeated it 3 times.	The client repeated it three times.	
These are 4 concepts that mean the same.	These are four concepts that mean the same.	
She is the only 1 who is well prepared.	She is the only one who is well prepared.	
The client has missed 2 or 3 sessions this semester.	The client has missed two or three sessions this semester.	
After 5 imitated responses, I will fade modeling.	After five imitated responses, I will fade modeling.	*Five* or *eight* is not in comparison with number 10 or above.
I will use 8 items for training.	I will use eight items for training.	
He got a 0 on the test.	He got a zero on the test.	The numbers *zero* and *one* in most (but not all) cases
Still, 1 response was wrong.	Still, one response was wrong. (*but*, Only 1 out of 15 was wrong.)	
Do not write a 1-sentence paragraph.	Do not write a one-sentence paragraph.	
One 5th of the class was absent today. 1/5th of the class was absent today.	One fifth of the class was absent today.	Common fractions *Note:* The second wrong example also starts the sentence with a number, another violation.
You need a 2/3 majority.	You need a two-thirds majority.	
The 4th of July was a hot day.	The Fourth of July was a hot day.	Traditionally expressed only in words
The 10 Commandments are well known.	The Ten Commandments are well known.	

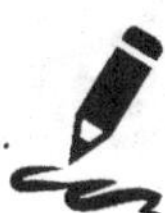

B.4.26b. Write Out in Words Numbers Below 10 in Specified Contexts

Incorrect	Write Correctly
At any one time, 4 to 5 students can observe the sessions.	
The instructor repeated it 4 times.	
These 5 terms have similar meanings.	
He is the only 1 who can be trusted.	
I used 6 stimuli on my probe list.	
It is no fun having 0-degree temperature.	
Today, 1/4th of the class is absent.	
The 12th Night is a play by Shakespeare.	
The original 12 Apostles were the disciples of Jesus.	

B.4.27a. Write Out in Words Any Number That Begins a Sentence

- Do not begin a sentence with a numeral.
- Apply this rule to titles and headings as well.

Incorrect	Correct	Note
5 children were tested.	Five children were tested.	No sentence starts with a number written in numerals.
75 clinicians attended the workshop.	Seventy-five clinicians attended the workshop.	
15% of the schoolchildren have some form of communicative disorder.	Fifteen percent of the schoolchildren have some form of communicative disorder.	
99 Ways to Get A Grades	Ninety-nine Ways to Get A Grades	Article title

B.4.28a. Combine Words and Numerals in Specified Contexts

Combine words and numerals to express

- large numbers (million and more)
- back-to-back modifiers

Incorrect	Correct	Note
Special education needs five billion dollars.	Special education needs $5 billion.	Large numbers
The population is at least five million.	The population is at least 5 million.	
We have two two-way mirrors. We have 2 2-way mirrors.	We have 2 two-way mirrors. or We have two 2-way mirrors.	Back-to-back numerical modifiers
We selected 6 9-year-olds for the study.	We selected six 9-year-olds for the study.	
I had the speech rated on 2 5-point scales.	I had the speech rated on two 5-point scales.	
Check the 1st 12 entries in the index.	Check the first 12 entries in the index.	

B.4.27b. Write Out in Words Any Number That Begins a Sentence

Incorrect	Write Correctly
9 phonemes will be trained.	
39th percentile is not too impressive.	
37 children will be screened.	
80% probe response rate did not meet the criterion.	
29 Methods of Stuttering Treatment [A paper]	

B.4.28b. Combine Words and Numerals in Specified Contexts

Incorrect	Write Correctly
You cannot really see seven million people at one time!	
The city has only two two-way streets.	
Our research included 7 2-year-olds.	
Use 3 7-point scales for reliability.	
Check the 1st 4 items on the menu.	
The city has a budget of ten million dollars.	

Reference Citations Within the Text

B.4.29a. Cite the Author's Last Name and Year or Years of Publication in the Text

Incorrect	Correct	Note
In her study of heavyweight champions, Jane Byson found that . . .	In her study of heavyweight champions, Byson (2021) found that . . .	When the author's name is part of the narration, place the year in parentheses. Only the last name.
Ticklishson stated that humor is good medicine (2022).	Ticklishson (2022) stated that humor is good medicine.	Type the year immediately after the name.
Byson (2019) found that the reaction time of his opponents was sluggish. . . . Byson (2019) also found that . . .	Byson (2019) found that the reaction time of his opponents was sluggish. . . . Byson also found that . . .	Omit the year when the same study is referred to again in the same paragraph and cannot be confused with another.
A study suggested that boxing causes brain damage; Hali, 2019	A study suggested that boxing causes brain damage (Hali, 2019).	When the name and the year are not in the narrative, both should be within parentheses.
In (2016), MacVinro reported that playing tennis sharpens the tongue.	In 2016, MacVinro reported that playing tennis sharpens the tongue.	A year that is a part of the narration should not be in parentheses.
Nemson, Jr. (2021) did the study.	Nemson (2021) did the study.	In the text, omit such name-suffixes as *Jr.* or *III.* Add them in the reference list.
Patterson's study (2014, October) included a small sample.	Patterson's study (2014) included a small sample.	In the text, do not cite the month even if it is cited in the reference list.
Russell in 1921 and 2005 contended that words do not carry meaning.	Russell (1921/2005) contended that words do not carry meaning.	First published in 1921 and reprinted in 2005; see B.4.57a on referencing such works.

B.4.30a. Cite Both Names in the Text When a Work Has Two Authors

Incorrect	Correct in Text	Note
Tang et al. (2013) found that college courses are incomprehensible.	Tang and Lagassi (2013) found that college courses are incomprehensible.	Cite both the authors in the first and all subsequent text citations. Use the conjunction *and.*
Evidence suggests that plagiarism is common on campuses (True et al., 2021).	Evidence suggests that plagiarism is common on campuses (True & Crew, 2022).	Cite both names in the first as well as all subsequent parenthetical constructions. Use the ampersand (&).

Reference Citations Within the Text

B.4.29b. Cite the Author's Last Name and Year or Years of Publication in the Text

Incorrect	Write Correctly
June Jinkinson (2019) stated that . . .	
In (2018), Torkinson reported that . . .	
Jasperson's study has shown that . . . (2011).	
Research shows that bilingualism is enriching; Fung, 2016.	
Packman III (2015) questioned the validity of such claims.	
Nunez completed the study (2014, June).	
Skinner in 1975 and 2003 stated that the concept of a free person is a myth.	

B.4.30b. Cite Both Names in the Text When a Work Has Two Authors

Reference Information	Write a Sentence Using the Information
1. Authors: Cheng and Tang Year: 2021 Study on: elimination of phonological processes. Results: Only some processes were eliminated.	1. Begin the sentence with the reference.
2. Authors: Haniff and Chwe Year: 2022 Study on: incidence of stuttering in general population Result: about 1%	2. End the sentence with the names in parentheses.

B.4.31a. Cite Works With Three or More Authors With Only the First Author

- Even on first citation, cite only the first author.
- Add "et al." to the first author's name (without quotation marks) and continue to cite the same way throughout the paper.

Incorrect	Correct	Parenthetical
In a study on head injury, Hali, Byson, and Tedson (2016) found that . . . (*first citation*)	In a study on head injury, Hali et al. (2016) found that . . . (*first and all subsequent narrative citations*)	It was reported that . . . (Hali et al., 2016). (*First and all parenthetical citations*)
In their study on vocal nodules, Lordon, Fontana, Tanseko, Pendl, and Tavratino (2015) discovered that . . . (*first citation*)	In their study on vocal nodules, Lordon et al. (2015) discovered that . . . (*first and all subsequent narrative citations*)	A study reported that . . . (Lordon et al., 2015). (*first and all subsequent parenthetical citations*)

B.4.31b. Cite Works With Three or More Authors With Only the First Author

Show the first and one subsequent citation.

Reference Information	Write a Sentence Using the Information
1. Authors: Shanker, Lee, Samuelson, and Mistry Year: 2020 Study: new surgical methods of closing the complete palatal cleft Results: favorable	1. Begin the sentence with the name; show first and subsequent citations.
2. Authors: Blinken, Gomez, and Pundit Year: 2019 Study: new methods of auditory masking Results: no improvement over existing methods	2. End the sentence showing the name within parentheses.

B.4.32a. Distinguish Works of Multiple Authors Published in the Same Year

- If two studies published in the same year with a different combination of three or more authors have the same first author, then cite all names if necessary; or cite as many names as needed to distinguish the two studies.

Incorrect	Correct	Note
Lordon et al. (2012) have concluded that . . . *(This study had four authors: Lordon, Fontana, Tanseko, and Pendl)* Lordon et al. (2012) also have concluded that . . . *(A different study published in the same year that had a different combination of four authors: Lordon, Fontana, Tanseko, and Jensen)*	Lordon, Fontana, Tanseko, and Pendl (2012) showed that . . . Lordon, Fontana, Tanseko, and Pendl (2012) have concluded that . . . *(All names of this study cited each time)* Lordon, Fontana, Tanseko, and Jensen (2012) also reported that . . . Lordon, Fontana, Tanseko, and Jensen (2012) also have concluded that . . . *(All names of this other study also cited each time)*	The four names of each of the two studies are cited all the time to distinguish the two studies. If not, the two studies would be confused as they both abbreviate to Lordon et al. (2012).
Tinsonn et al. (2005) have found no significant difference. *(This study had seven authors: Tinsonn, Fung, Haniff, Chwe, Boonthenthorpe, Alvarado, and Smith)* Tinsonn et al. (2005) did not find the method effective. *(This study had six authors: Tinsonn, Fung, Mendoza, Kumar, Azevedo, and Alfonso)*	Tinsonn, Fung, et al. (2005) have found no significant difference. Tinsonn, Fung, Mendoza, et al. (2005) did not find the method effective.	The two studies had multiple authors in different combination, published in the same year. The addition of a third name distinguishes the two studies. A comma is added to the last name (before et al.) because of multiple names.

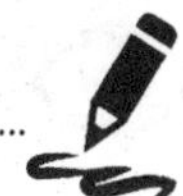

B.4.32b. Distinguish Works of Multiple Authors Published in the Same Year

- Write the names of as many authors as needed to distinguish the two studies.

Reference Information	Write a Sentence Using the Information
1. Authors: Rodriguez, Ford, Williams, Johnson, and Benson Year: 2017 Study: modeling target responses Result: useful	1.
2. Authors: Rodriguez, Ford, Williams, Bennet, Bickley, and Shekar Year: 2017 Study: Incidence of stuttering Results: 1% in the general population	2.

B.4.33a. Join Multiple Author Names With the Conjunction *and* or the Ampersand

- Join the author names with *and* when the citation is part of the narrative.
- Join the author names with & (ampersand) when the citation is in parentheses.

Incorrect	Correct	Note
A study of Hecker & Donnors (2003) showed that . . .	A survey of Hecker and Donnors (2003) showed that . . .	The names are a part of the narrative. Conjunction *and* is correct.
Spitting on the field increases the number of hits (Rosen and Tanseko, 2008).	Spitting on the field increases the number of hits (Rosen & Tanseko, 2008).	The names are in parentheses. The ampersand is correct.

B.4.34a. Distinguish the Different First Authors With the Same Surname

- If two or more first authors have the same surname listed in the reference list, add the initials to the first surname even in the text citation.
- Follow this rule even if the years of publication are different.

Within the Text	In the Reference List	Note
Studies of F. Pomaville (2022) and M. Pomaville and Pomaville (2015) reveal that . . .	Pomaville, F. (2022). *Assessment of communication disorders in children*. Plural Publishing. Pomaville, M., & Pomaville, K. (2015). A review of voice assessment procedures. *Journal of Voice, 28,* 56–69.	Three different authors with the same surname. In the case of paired authors, the initials are added only to the first author in the text.

B.4.33b. Join Multiple Author Names With the Conjunction *and* or the Ampersand

Reference Information	Write a Sentence Using the Information
1. Part of narration Authors: Gimmick and Himmick Year: 2000 Study: the relation between screaming and vocal nodules Results: positive relation	1.
2. Citation in parentheses Authors: Byson and Lyson Year: 1992 Study: programming maintenance Results: possible to program maintenance	2.

B.4.34b. Distinguish the Different First Authors With the Same Surname

In the Reference List	Write a Text Sentence
Maul, M. (2016). *Assessment of autistic children.* Mayfair Press. Maul, O., & Maul, Q. (2015). Treatment of autistic children. *Journal of Autism, 28*, 56–69.	*Note:* Include both sources in your sentence.

B.4.35a. Cite Multiple Works of the Same Author in a Temporally Ascending Order

- **Do not** use the conjunction *and* before the final year (2005, 2007, 2015; but **not**, 2005, 2007, *and* 2015).
- Note that *in press* has no year attached to it.

Incorrect	Correct	Note
Studies show that the more exciting the game, the greater is the injury to vocal folds (Fontana, 1997, 1999, and in press 2022).	Studies show that the more exciting the game, the greater is the injury to vocal folds (Fontana 1997, 1999, 2001, in press).	The earliest publication is cited first; the *in press* citation is always the most recent, hence the last, and because it is not yet published, no year is attached.
Studies of Tonseko and Travlatinova (2001, 1999, 1997, 1996) have shown that verbal abuse is a common locker room strategy.	Studies of Tonseko and Travlatinova (1996, 1997, 1999, 2001) have shown that verbal abuse is a common locker room strategy.	The incorrect versions are in the descending temporal order of publication.
Data suggest that yells that induce vocal nodules excite the players (Rosery & Ruthery, 2001; 1995; 1998).	Data suggest that yells that induce vocal nodules excite the players (Rosery & Ruthery, 1995, 1998, 2001).	The correct versions show references in parentheses in the ascending order, separated by a comma, not a semicolon.

B.4.36a. Attach Alphabetical Suffixes to the Same Author's Multiple Publications in the Same Year

- Repeat the year; do not affix a, b, c, and so forth to year typed only once (2015a, 2015b, 2015c; but **not** 2015a, b, c).
- In assigning a, b, c, and so forth to studies published in the same year, use the alphabetical order of the first word of titles of articles.

Incorrect	Correct	Note
Several studies by Johnson (2000-1, 2000-2, 2000-3, in press-a, in press-2 have shown that . . .	• Several studies (Johnson, 2000a, 2000b, 2000c, in press-a, in press-b have shown that . . .	• Multiple *in press* entries also take -a, -b, -c, and so forth.
Ball game watching may increase the brain size (Fontana, 1988-1, 1988-2, 1991-1, 1999-2 in press-1, in press-2; Tanseko, 2015-1, 2015-2, 2016-1, 2016-2, in press-1, in press-2).	Ball game watching may increase the brain size (Fontana, 1988a, 1988b, 1991a, 1999b in press-a, in press-b; Tanseko, 2015a, 2015b, 2016a, 2016b, in press-a, in press-b).	• Multiple authors, each publishing multiple studies in each of the two years; references in parentheses.

B.4.35b. Cite Multiple Works of the Same Author in Temporally Ascending Order

Reference Information	Write a Sentence Using the Information
Author: McVinro Study: treatment of hoarse voice Studies published in: 2001, 1999, 2000, 1989	The author's name in narration. Include the author's name in your narration.
Authors: Moncure and Sincure Study: bilingual-bicultural issues Studies published in: 2002, 1996, 1989, 1999	The authors' name in parentheses Enclose the authors' names in parentheses.
Author: Foresight Study: future professional issues Studies published in: 2002, 2001, 1999, 1998, 1997	The author's name in parentheses Enclose the author's name in parentheses.

B.4.36b. Attach Alphabetical Suffixes to the Same Author's Multiple Publications in the Same Year

Reference Information	Write a Sentence Using the Information
Author: Sharp Study: advances in cochlear implants Published: four in 2002	Author's name in the narrative
Author: Bulltit Study: dysphagia assessment techniques Published: three in 1999, two in 2001 Author: Hiltit Study: dysphagia assessment techniques Published: two in 1989; two in 2001	Authors' and their publications in parentheses

B.4.37a. Within Parentheses, Arrange the Last Names of Multiple Authors in Alphabetical Order

- Use the last name of the first author to determine the alphabetical order.
- Separate each name with a semicolon.
- Do not type *and* or & before the last citation.

Incorrect	Correct	Note
(Zoom, 1999; Began, 2000; Push, 1998; Lord, 1997)	(Began, 2000; Lord, 1997; Push, 1998; Zoom, 1999)	Follow the alphabetical, not temporal, order.
(Push & Twink, 1999; Began & Quinn, 1990; Lord, Horde, & Board, 1985)	(Began & Quinn, 1990; Lord, Horde, & Board, 1985; Push & Twink, 1999)	The last name of the first author determines the order. An ampersand joins the multiple names.
(Benson, 1989; Dinson, 1992; Henson, 1990; and Nelson, 1986)	(Benson, 1989; Dinson, 1992; Henson, 1990; Nelson, 1986)	Omit *and* before the last entry.
(Bloodstein, 1987; Epstein, 1995; & Fonstein, 1990)	(Bloodstein, 1987; Epstein, 1995; Fonstein, 1990)	Omit the ampersand before the last entry.

B.4.38a. Cite Secondary Sources Sparingly and Correctly

- Secondary sources are books and articles that you found in a source other than the original.
- To maintain scholarly integrity, read the original sources (books, journal articles) and cite them to eliminate secondary citations.
- Cite no more than just a few unavoidable secondary sources that may be out of print, unavailable, or in languages you do not understand.

Correct	Note
Deepthought's classic study, as cited in Alvarado (1999), showed that . . . Deepthought's (1920) classic study, as cited in Alvarado (1999), showed that . . .	The date of the original study (*Deepthought's*, in this case) may not be available; but if available, it is cited. In either case, only the secondary source (Alvarado, 1999, in the example) is listed in the reference list.

B.4.37b. Within Parentheses, Arrange the Last Names of Multiple Authors in Alphabetical Order

Reference Information	Cite the Names Within Parentheses
Authors: Thompson, 1999 Johnson, 2001 Quinn, 2000	
Authors: Zonks and Gonks, 1998 Banks and Atkins, 1995 Atkins, 1990 Kinson, 2001	
Authors: Bayle, 1997 Timson, 1996 Xenon, 1998 Lyson, 2002	

B.4.38b. Cite Secondary Sources Sparingly and Correctly

Reference Information	Cite Correctly
Original study by: Kinkler Found in: Peakson, 2000	

B.4.39a. Cite Correctly the Works With No Author or an Anonymous Author

- In the text, cite the first few words of the title of an article, a book chapter, or a web page within double quotation marks and add the year.
- Italicize the title of a journal, book, or report.

In the Text	Note
The professional guidelines ("Best Practice," 2016) are clear.	This may be from a webpage.
Investment for young professionals (2017) is a useful book.	Book with no author. Place the book title in the author position in the reference list.
This is a frequently stated opinion (Anonymous, 2012).	*Anonymous* is treated like a name itself in the reference list.

B.4.39b. Cite Correctly the Works With No Author or an Anonymous Author

Sources	Write Correctly
New healthcare [a web article]	
Becoming a Clinician (2017) [a book.]	
Many believe in this view [Anonymous source, 2012]	

B.4.40a. Cite Correctly the Year of Publication in Parenthetical Text

In The Text	Note
The details may be found elsewhere (e.g., the U.S. Census Report, 2015, Table 5).	The year of publication is preceded and followed by a comma, not brackets.

B.4.41a. Cite Correctly the Specific Parts of a Source

- Occasionally, a chapter, a page, a figure, or a table in a source may be cited.
- The source is included in the reference list.

In The Text	Note
The latest statistics are of clinical concern (Brain Injury Association, 2016, p. 22).	*Page* is abbreviated to small p.
The reader is referred to another source (Freed, 2016, Chapter 5).	*Chapter*, *Table*, and *Figure* are not abbreviated.

B.4.40b. Cite Correctly the Year of Publication in Parenthetical Text

In the Text	Write Correctly
Write a sentence to include the following: The American Speech-Language-Hearing Association's Report on Reimbursement Year: 2017 Figure: 5	The citation is referenced in the reference list.

B.4.41b. Cite Correctly the Specific Parts of a Source

In the Text	Write Correctly
Write a sentence to include the following: Health and Human Services Year: 2014 Table: 7	
Write a sentence to include the following: Author: Skelton Year: 2017 Figure: 8-1	

Reference List

B.4.42. General Guidelines on Creating a Reference List

- Most students, professionals, and scientists search for research articles on academic research databases including MEDLINE, MEDLINE Plus, EBSCO, ERIC, Google Scholar, Linguistics and Language Behavior Abstracts (ProQuest), PsychInfo, PubMed, ScienceDirect, Cochrane Library (for systematic reviews of treatment research), and others depending on the topic of interest. These databases contain peer-reviewed journal articles that are critical for academic study and research. Such databases are generally trustworthy. Students and faculty at most universities and colleges may gain access to full-text articles on these databases by logging into them through their university library account.
- Scholarly articles and books generally depend on print sources, rather than internet-only sources. Exceptions include journals published only online and classic books and materials available online. Most print journals or their articles also have electronic versions, but you should cite the version you read.
- In a reference list,
  - include all that is cited and only what is cited in the text
  - arrange authors in an alphabetical order
  - use the author initials to alphabetize the entries with the same last names
  - treat "Anonymous" as though it is the author's name, and alphabetize
  - alphabetize the different corporate authors (e.g., American Psychological . . . before American Speech-Language-Hearing . . .)
  - alphabetize the works with no author by the first significant word of the title (ignore *a*, *an*, *the*, and so forth)
  - alphabetize a numeral that starts a title as though it is written in words, e.g., 100 [One hundred] precedes 10 [Ten]
  - double-space the entire list
  - format each paragraph with the hanging indent of 0.05 in.
  - omit the publisher's name when the same entity (an organization, association) wrote and published a book (e.g., the APA *Manual*); specify the DOI, if available
  - note that a *reference list* is attached to a paper, a book, or other form of writing, whereas a *bibliography* is a comprehensive list of publications on a topic and typically stands alone (not attached to any text)
- See B.4.62 and B.4.63 for referencing electronic sources on the web.
- The following pages sample different kinds of entries in a reference list. Consult the APA *Manual* for additional examples.

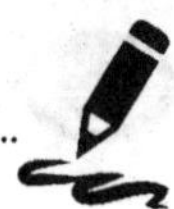

B.4.43a. Begin the Reference List on a New Page With a Centered Heading

References	
Able, T. K. (2020). *Children with autism: New directions in assessment and treatment* (4th ed.). Sapson Press.	Published book
Able, Q. T. (2012). Dream analysis in language therapy with 2-year-old children. *Journal of Dream Language, 35*(4), 55–95.	A journal article without DOI
Abur, D., Perkell, J. S., & Stepp, C. E. (2022). Impact of vocal effort on respiratory and articulatory kinematics. *Journal of Speech, Language, and Hearing Research, 65*(1), 1–4. https://doi.org/10.1044/2021_JSLHR-21-00513	A journal article with DOI
American Psychiatric Association. (2013). *Diagnostic and statistical manual of mental disorders* (5th ed.). https://doi.org/10.1176/appi.books.9780890425596	Author is the publisher.
American Speech-Language-Hearing Association. (n.d.). Frequently asked questions: Obtaining reimbursement for stuttering treatment. https://www.asha.org/practice/reimbursement/private-plans/reimb_stutter_trtmnt/	From a professional organization's webpage
Centers for Disease Control and Prevention. (2022, January 20). *CDC releases update maps of America's high levels of inactivity* [Press release]. https://www.cdc.gov/media/releases/2022/p0120-inactivity-map.html	A press release; no retrieval date necessary.
18 Famous people who stutter. Stuttering Foundation. https://www.stutteringhelp.org/sites/default/files/FamousPeople.pdf	No author article title alphabetized as Eighteen
Hale, L. S. (2017). The effects of medication on communication in older adulthood. In R. H. Hull (Ed.), *Communication disorders in aging* (pp. 155–178). Plural Publishing.	A chapter in an edited book
Merriam-Webster. (n.d.). Communication. In *Merriam-Webster.com dictionary.* Retrieved February 10, 2022, from https://www.merriam-webster.com/	Dictionary entry with no date (n.d)
National Institute on Deafness and Other Communication Disorders. (n.d.). *Pendred syndrome.* Retrieved January 27, 2022, from https://www.nidcd.nih.gov/health/pendred-syndrome	From a government agency's webpage
National Institute of Mental Health. (2015, April 14). *"Follow That Cell" prize winners* [Video]. YouTube. https://www.youtube.com/watch?v=lwvsvIPZLUI	YouTube posting from a government agency.
Remnnick, D. (Host) (2022, January 21). *The trials of a whistle blower* [Audio podcast]. *New Yorker.* https://www.newyorker.com/podcast/the-new-yorker-radio-hour/the-trials-of-a-whistle-blower	An audio podcast
World Health Organization. (2019). International statistical classification of disorders and related health problems (11th ed.). https://icd.who.int/	The same author and publisher.
Your COVID-19 vaccination. (2021, November 3). Centers for Disease Control and Prevention. https://www.cdc.gov/coronavirus/2019-ncov/vaccines/your-vaccination.html	Title of a work with no author, alphabetized.

B.4.43b. Begin the Reference List on a New Page With a Centered Heading

Write the word *References* in its correct position. Invent the necessary information to correctly write the reference for specified entry categories. Alphabetize your list.

	A book with two authors
	A single author's chapter in a book with one editor
	Print version of a journal article, two authors, with DOI
	A book written by an organization
	From a professional organization's webpage
	A press release; frequently updated
	A chapter in an edited book
	Dictionary with no date (n.d.)
	From a government agency's webpage
	YouTube posting from a government agency
	An audio podcast
	A publication with no author

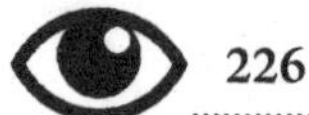

B.4.44a. In the Reference List, Arrange Authors in Alphabetical Order

- Use the last name to determine the alphabetical order.
- Alphabetize the names of multiple authors by the surname of the first author.
- Alphabetize names letter by letter but exclude the initials.
- Arrange prefixes in their strict alphabetical order. Ignore an apostrophe attached to a prefix (M')
- Consult the biographical section of *Merriam-Webster's* online dictionary Biographical Names section to find the order in which surnames with articles and prepositions are arranged (names with *de*, *la*, *du*, *von*, etc.).
- When listing several works by the same author, but some with and some without coauthors, start with those works that do not have coauthors.

Incorrect	Correct	Note
McNeil, A. S. (2010) Macmillan, J. J. (2008)	Macmillan, J. J. (2008) McNeil, A. S. (2010)	*Mac* precedes *Mc*
Thomson, A. B. (2016) Thomas, Z. X. (2015)	Thomas, Z. X. (2015) Thomson, A. B. (2016)	Alphabetized letter by letter. Ignore the initials.
Tonseko, K. J., & Fontana, P. J. (2001) Tonseko, K. J., & Lordon, T. P. (2017) Tonseko, K. J. (2013)	Tonseko, K. J. (2013) Tonseko, K. J., & Fontana, P. J. (2001) Tonseko, K. J., & Lordon, T. P. (2017)	Enter the single author first. Alphabetize the second authors, too: *Tonseko & Fontana* before *Tonseko & Lordon*.

B.4.45a. Arrange Multiple Works of the Same Single Author From the Earliest to the Latest Year

Incorrect	Correct	Note
Able, P. J. (2017) Able, P. J. (1992) Able, P. J. (1989)	Able, P. J. (1989) Able, P. J. (1992) Able, P. J. (2017)	For each single author, arrange the works from the earliest to the latest year.
Benson, L. S. (2016) Benson, L. S. (2008) Benson, L. S. (2002)	Benson, L. S. (2002) Benson, L. S. (2008) Benson, L. S. (2016)	

B.4.44b. In the Reference List, Arrange Authors in Alphabetical Order

Reference Information	Arrange the Names Alphabetically
McMinnan, L. D., 2010 McDonald, U. G., 2015 McFarrin, M. P., 2012 Van Riper, C., 1975 Axelrod, A. K., 2016 Herbert, B. H., 2009 Hernadez, N. K., 2013 Alvarado, B. C., 2014 von Kirk, D., 2011 de Klerk, Q. Q., 2017	

B.4.45b. Arrange Multiple Works of the Same Single Author From the Earliest to the Latest Year

Reference Information	Arrange the Names in the Correct Order
Larson, K. (2016) Larson, K. (2007) Larson, K. (2002)	
McDonald, P. (2014) McDonald, P. (2001) McDonald, P. (2007)	

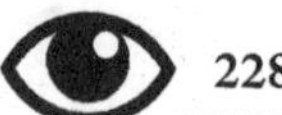

B.4.46a. Alphabetize the Titles of Several Works of the Same Author Published in the Same Year

- Ignore the articles *a* and *the* at the beginning of the title.
- Attach the lowercase letters a, b, c, and so forth, to the year of publication.

Incorrect	Correct	Note
Lagassi, A. R. (2015a). Problems of clay courts. Lagassi, A. R. (2015b). Advantages of short-handled rackets.	Lagassi, A. R. (2015a). Advantages of short-handled rackets. Lagassi, A. R. (2015b). Problems of clay courts.	The first word of the title is used to alphabetize: *Advantages* precedes *Problems.*
Massood, P. T. (2010a). Some advantages of the circular paper clip. Massood, P. T. (2010b). The case of the missing paper clip.	Massood, P. T. (2010a). The case of the missing paper clip. Massood, P. T. (2010b). Some advantages of the circular paper clip.	The article *The* is ignored in arranging these two entries.

B.4.47a. Arrange the Multiple Works of the Same Author Published in Different Years in Temporally Ascending Order

Incorrect	Correct	Note
Nelson, B. D. (2001). AIDS in the modern world. Nelson, B. D. (1998). Beads around the neck. Nelson, B. D. (2002). Lost in theories.	Nelson, B. D. (1998). Beads around the neck. Nelson, B. D. (2001). AIDS in the modern world. Nelson, B. D. (2002). Lost in theories.	The titles are not alphabetized.

B.4.48a. Alphabetize the Different Authors With the Same Last Name According to Their Initials

Incorrect	Correct	Note
Able, Q. T. (1993) Able, A. A. (1982)	Able, A. A. (1982) Able, Q. T. (1993)	The year of publication does not matter.
Tavratinova, S. N. (1987) Tavratinova, B. D. (1993)	Tavratinova, B. D. (1993) Tavratinova, S. N. (1987)	

B.4.46b. Alphabetize the Titles of Several Works of the Same Author Published in the Same Year

Reference Information	Alphabetize According to the Titles
Belwae, T. P. (1989a). A potential explanation of muddy football fields. Belwae, T. P. (1989b). Crashing and winning: The cultural underpinnings of football.	
Cisnero, S. M. (1990a). Cities in decay: An agenda for rebuilding American cities. Cisnero, S. M. (1990b). Banking on the neighborhood.	

B.4.47b. Arrange the Multiple Works of the Same Author Published in Different Years in Temporally Ascending Order

Incorrect	Arrange Correctly
Nayyar, C. D. (2001). All can learn. Nayyar, C. D. (1998). Help for the homeless. Nayyar, C. D. (2002). Polish the self-image.	

B.4.48b. Alphabetize the Different Authors With the Same Last Name According to Their Initials

Reference Information	Alphabetize According to the Initials
Nelson, Z. T. (2016) Nelson, B. S. (2013) Nelson, A. P. (2015)	
Ramig, L. T. (2017) Ramig, C. C. (2011) Ramig, B. D. (2015)	

B.4.49a. Format Each Entry in the Reference List With a Hanging Indent of Five Spaces

- Use the word processor's default setting for hanging indents.
- Note that each entry is treated as a separate paragraph with its hanging indent.

Incorrect	Correct	Note

Lagassi, A. R. (1991a).
Advantages of short-handled
rackets. *Journal of Rackets, 4,*
55–90.
Lagassi, A. R. (1991b).
Problems of clay courts. The
Racket Press.
	Lagassi, A. R. (1991a).
	     Advantages of short-handled
	     rackets. *Journal of Rackets, 4,*
	     55–90.
	Lagassi, A. R. (1991b).
	     Problems of clay courts. The
	     Racket Press.
		When you select the *hanging indent* feature in your word processor, the first line of each entry is flush left, and the second and subsequent lines of each entry are indented.

B.4.50a. Use the Specified Abbreviations in Reference Lists

- Note that in reference lists, most of the abbreviations are placed within parentheses and may include other elements (e.g., number of pages, report, edition, etc.).

Abbreviation	For	Note
(2nd ed.)	second edition	Lowercase abbreviations
(p.) or (pp.)	page (pages)	
(n.d.)	no date	
(Vol.) or (Vols.)	Volume or Volumes	Uppercase abbreviations
(Ed.) or (Eds.)	Editor or Editors	
(Trans.)	Translator or Translators	
(Rev. ed.)	Revised edition	
(No.)	Number	
(Pt.)	Part	
(Rep.)	Report	
(Tech.)	(Technical)	
(Suppl.)	Supplement	

B.4.49b. Format Each Entry in the Reference List With a Hanging Indent of Five Spaces

Invent a journal name, volume number, and page numbers for both the references.

Incorrect	Rewrite Correctly
Sharma, P. K. (1989). Mothers teach language to their children. Tackle, K. K. (1990). Tackle football and the moral fiber.	

B.4.50b. Use the Specified Abbreviations in Reference Lists

Unabbreviated	Write the Correct Abbreviation
Edition	
Revised edition	
Second edition	
Editor (Editors)	
Translator(s)	
Page (pages)	
Volume	
Number	
Part	
Report	
Technical	
Supplement	
No date	

Selected Examples of References

Printed Journal Articles

B.4.51. Overview of Referencing Printed Journal Articles

- Enter one space between author initials, after the last initial, before starting the article title, and before the journal name.
- Type a comma after the last initial of the first author and join the names of two authors with an ampersand (&); type a period after the year in parentheses.
- Reference a maximum of 20 authors in the reference list if the work has more than 21 authors; note that no conjunction *and* or the ampersand *&* connect any authors in this case; see B.4.53a for the format.
- Capitalize all important words of the journal name; do not abbreviate it; italicize the journal name and the volume number (but no *volume* or its abbreviation).
- Enter the issue number, if available, in parentheses with no space after the volume number; use roman font, not the italics used for the volume number.
- Type "Advance online publication" without the quote marks if the source is published ahead of print; volume, issue, or page numbers may be unavailable, but copy the entire URL, which will include the DOI or a PubMed number that ASHA journals use; see B.4.63 for examples.
- Enter the page number or numbers as the last entry without *p.* or *pp.*; end the entry with a period; do not italicize the page numbers.
- Write "in press" without the quotation marks for articles in press.
- If a publication has no date, type n.d. in parentheses instead of the year of publication.
- Give the month (for monthlies) or month and date (for dailies) after the year in parentheses.
- Include the Digital Object Identifier (DOI) number, if available; copy the entire URL (beginning with https://) exactly, with no period at the end; with DOI, no additional retrieval information is needed.
- Note that several examples with no full DOI numbers are constructed to illustrate the different elements of an entry; do not try to find them.

B.4.52a. Use the Correct Format to Reference Printed Journal Articles

Correct	Note
American Speech-Language-Hearing Association. (n.d.). Prohibitions against discrimination under ASHA's Code of Ethics and enforcement by the Board of Ethics. https://www.asha.org/practice/ethics/prohibitions-against-discrimination-under-asha-code-of-ethics/	(n.d.) replaces the year when a publication date is unknown. Note how certain proper nouns are capitalized; there is no DOI, so give the web address.
Capriotti, M. R., & Donaldson, J. M. (2022). "Why don't behavior analysts do something?" Behavior analysts' historical, present, and potential future actions on sexual gender minority issues. *Journal of Applied Behavior Analysis*, *55*(1), 19–39. https://doi.10.1002/jaba.884	Even though all DOIs start with the numeral 10, they are unique to each article and its publisher; copy it exactly. For more information, visit http://www.doi.org/
McVenro, D. (2022). The relation between umpire judgments and player verbal outbursts. *American Sportsman*, *520*, 1230–1240.	Example of an article published in a monthly magazine. No DOI.
Polka, L., Masapollo, M., & Menard, L. (2022). Setting the stage for speech production: Infants prefer listening to speech sound with infant vocal resonances. *Journal of Speech, Language, and Hearing Research*, *65*(1), 109–120. https://doi.org/10.1044/2021_JSLHR-21-00412	Do not abbreviate the journal name; capitalize all major words. Add the issue number within parentheses in roman font after the italicized volume number; no space separates the volume and issue numbers.
Stark, B. C., & Cofoid, C. (2022). Task-specific iconic gesturing during spoken discourse in aphasia. *American Journal of Speech-Language Pathology*, *31*(1), 30–47. https://doi.org/10.1044/2021_AJSLP-20-00271	Italicize only the journal name and volume number, not the issue number. Give the page numbers after the *volume*(issue) numbers.
Tomlinson, B., & Godson, T. (in press). Nutty theories in naughty disciplines. *Journals of Theoretical Speculations*.	You will not find other reference elements for an article in the process of publication.
Onque, R., & Roland, D. (2022). New Covid variant: What we know about the BA.2 Omicron strain. *The Wall Street Journal*. https://www.wsj.com/articles/what-we-know-about-the-ba-2-omicron-variant-11643300997	A newspaper article. Italicize the newspaper name. Give the web address (not a DOI).
Pham, U., Skogseid, I. M., Pripp, A. H., Bøen, E., & Toft, M. (2021). Impulsivity in Parkinson's disease patients treated with subthalamic nucleus deep brain stimulation—An exploratory study. *PLOS ONE*, *16*(3). Article e0248568. https://doi.org/10.1371/journal.pone.0248568	Cite the eLocator when available. Some journals give an article number or an eLocator.

Printed Journal Articles

B.4.52b. Use the Correct Format to Reference Printed Journal Articles

Reference Information	Correctly Write the References
Author: P. E. Turkeltaub Year: 2015 Article Title: Brain stimulation and the role of the right hemisphere in aphasia recovery Journal: *Current Neurology and Neuroscience Reports* Volume: 15 Pages: 72–79 DOI:10.1007/s11910-015-0593-6	*Note:* Both DOI and doi are used by different sources.
Author: S. L. Nunez Year: in press Article Title: Models of counseling in speech and hearing Journal: *American Journal of Speech-Language Pathology*	
Authors: C. C. Woo, and M. Leon Year: 2013 Article Title: Environmental enrichment as treatment for autism. Journal: *Behavioral Neuroscience* Volume: 127 Issue number: 4 Pages: 487–497	

B.4.53a. Arrange Correctly the Articles With Multiple Authors

- Include all author names up to 20 authors of a multi-authored work.
- Include the first 19 names, enter an ellipsis mark (. . .), and then add the very last author name of a work that contains 21 or more authors.
- The reference list will not contain more than 20 author names.

Correct	Note
Raj, R. J. (1959).	A single author
Hellbent, H. B., & Heavenbound, L. T. (2020).	Two authors
Moll, D., Black, K., Ball, A., Dole, B., White, T., Jha, A., Neal, P., Ford, J., Lu, C., Board, N., Lee, L., Nerd, M., Jen, S., Wu, L., Higgins, H., Piggins, P., Cheng, R., Roy, B., Joseph, J., . . . Murthy, M. (2021).	A paper with 21 or more authors. Enter the first **19** authors, and then insert an ellipsis mark (. . .), and add the **very last** author's name of the work. Do not add *et al.* or the ampersand (&). Note that Murthy is not the 21st author; she is the very last author.

B.4.54a. Reference Correctly the Different Types of Journal Publications

- Note that reference entry examples for many other types of periodical publications are given throughout this section.

Correct	Note
Broadhead, K. D. (Ed.). (2001). Ineffective but popular stuttering therapies [Special issue]. *Journal of Stuttering Therapy, 55*(7). https://doi.org/xxxxx	Referencing an entire [Special issue] of a journal with the editor's name. Note the brackets (not parentheses) and the absence of page numbers.
Deshmukh, S. R., Holmes, J., & Cardno, A. (2018). Art therapy for people with dementia. *Cochrane Database of Systematic Reviews*. https://doi.org/10.1002/14651858.CD011073.pub2	A systematic review article published by the Cochrane Database. Retrieval information copied from the site.
Moyer, M. W. (2022). Schooled in lies. *Scientific American, 326*(2), 34–39. https://doi.org/10.1038/scientificamerican0222-34	A magazine article.
Ireland, M., & Conrad, B. J. (2016). Evaluation and eligibility for speech-language services in schools. *Perspectives of the ASHA Special Interest Groups, SIG 16,* 1(Pt. 4), 78–90. https://doi.org/10.xxxx	ASHA SIG print publication. Give DOI if available.
Hatcher, A., Frost, K., Weiler, B., & Bland, L. (2022). A survey of speech-language pathologists' perceptions of telepractice pre- and posttraining during the COVID-19 pandemic. *Perspectives of the ASHA Special Interest Groups, SIG 18.* Advance online publication. https://doi.org/10.1044/2021_PERSP-21-00196	Electronic publication ahead of the print issue.

B.4.53b. Arrange Correctly the Articles With Multiple Authors

- In place of DOI, write: https://doi.org/10.xxxx

Reference Information	Correctly Write the References
Authors: B. D. Jasper and K. D. Master Year: 2001 Article: Communicative intents Journal: *Intuitive Language Pathology, 190,* 15–35.	
Authors: T. T. Ladd, C. Badd, S. Lode, L. Jode, K., Node, and Z. Goad Year: 2002 Article: Do not believe in it. Journal: *Journal of Metaphysics, 50,* 30–40.	*Hint:* Six authors
Authors: D. Monsen, D. Benson, N. Shankar, B. Banerjee, K. Johnson, A. Nonsense, G. Dollard, T. Ladd, C. Badd, S. Lode, M. Node, B. Miller, S. Terror, Z. Goad, T. Caam, B. Lee, S. Win, T. Lose, J. Joy, R. Reid, P. Pun, D. Down, Q. Upman, I. Ivan, O. Oza, U. Urs, V. Sharp Year: 2000 Article: Yawning as treatment for voice disorders Journal: *Journal of Voice and Communication Disorders, 52,* 30–60.	*Hint:* More than 21 authors

B.4.54b. Reference Correctly the Different Types of Journal Publications

Reference Information	Correctly Write the References
Editor: M. K. Kim Year: 2015 Special issue: Therapies that work *Journal of Stuttering Therapy, 75.*	
Author: J. D. Jogg Year: 2017 A supplement to a journal: A study on morphologic learning. *Journal of Language* vol. 10, Supplement 5, pp. 2–45.	
Roberts, S. R. Year: (2022). Article: COVID and los of learning Magazine: *Science for Everyone, 12*(2), 15-25	
England, U. K., & Ireland, N. I. (2021). Vaccination rates in Eastern Europe. Journal: European Scientist, volume 10, pages 20-35 ePublication ahead of print	

Magazines and Newspaper Articles

B.4.55a. Reference Correctly the Publications From Magazines and Newspapers

Correct	Note
Kraft, J. P. (2001, September 10). America's drug war. *Newsweek*, 35–45.	A weekly magazine with no volume number.
Local therapist offers new treatment for autism. (2021, September 9). *Los Angeles Times*, p. B10. Retrieved from http://www.xxxxxx	Newspaper articles with no author. In the reference list, alphabetize according to the first significant word. Add the retrieval information if read online. In the text, cite a short title with the year (e.g., "Local therapist, 2001"); use double quotation marks.
New ways of treating heart disease. (2022, December 15). *The Fresno Bee*, pp. C5, C7, C9–11.	
Thomson, B. L. (2002, Fall). State legislature renews the licensure law. *CSHA*, 5–6.	Article in a newsletter with an author. If no author, alphabetize the title.

Abstracts

B.4.56a. Reference Correctly the Article Abstracts Used as the Primary Source

- The writer may have read only an abstract, which needs to be referenced (as in a database that contains only abstracts).
- The printed source may publish only an abstract of articles (as most convention programs do).

Correct	Note
Kemer, J. J. (2011, August 29). Preventing aspiration [Abstract]. *ASHA Leader*, *6*(15), 59.	The word *Abstract* in brackets (not italicized). The year is followed by the month and date.
Kimm, T. T., & Limm, P. P. (2020). Treatment of aphasia: A review [Abstract]. *Society for Aphasia Abstracts*, *10*, 59.	Example of a printed abstract source that the writer consulted.
Knudsen, O. O. (2019). Cognitive processes as ghosts of neuroscience. *Mexican Journal of Behavior Science*, *5*, 55. Abstract retrieved from https://www.xxxxxx	Example of an abstract obtained from an electronic database. Copy the exact URL.

Magazines and Newspaper Articles

B.4.55b. Reference Correctly the Publications From Magazines and Newspapers

Reference Information	Correctly Write the References
Author: Biff, L. P. Date: 2021, November 15 Article: School violence is declining Published in: *Time* (weekly) Pages: 10–15	
Article: The clinic in town saves life Date: 2019, July 10 Published in: *New York Times* (daily) Page: B20	
Zinson, L. L. (2015). Licensure laws are about to sunset in several states. Date: 2015, Winter Published in: *Speech and Hearing* (newsletter) Page: 20	

Abstracts

B.4.56b. Reference Correctly the Article Abstracts Used as the Primary Source

Incorrect	Correctly Write the References
Author: Zen, B. B.; Date: 2015, August 29 Article presented: Preventing stuttering Form: Abstract; Published in: *ASHA Leader*; *Volume 8*, issue 15, page 20	
Johns, T. T., & Hams, P. P.; Year: 2020 Article: Treatment of autism; Abstract Published in: *Association for Autism Abstracts; volume 12*, page 90	
Author: Kompleks, B. O.; year 2017 Article: Stuttering is awfully complex. Journal: *British Journal of Communication*; *volume 75*, pages 45–55. Abstract Retrieved from http://www.xxxxxx	

Books and Book Chapters

B.4.57a. Authored Books in Reference Lists

- Italicize the title of the book. Capitalize only the first letter of the title and subtitle.
- Type the abbreviated word *Jr.* after the last initial, if applicable.
- Type the abbreviated edition number (e.g., 2nd ed.) or the words "Rev. ed." (for *revised edition*; without quotation marks) after the title and place within parentheses.
- Type the publishing company's name exactly as it appears in the book being referenced.
- For books written and published by the same entity (e.g., corporations or associations), omit the publisher's name.
- For books originally published in one year and reprinted or reissued later by another publisher, give both years, and specify both publishers.

Correct	Note
American Psychological Association. (2020). *Publication manual of the American Psychological Association* (7th ed.). https://doi .org/10.1037/0000165-000	The publisher and the author are the same, so no need to specify the publisher. Most books do not have a DOI; include if available.
Boczquats, N. S. (2020). *Oceanography and communication: A new frontier.* Blue Press.	One space separates the year and the title and the title and the publisher.
Carpenter, C., & Taylor, T. (2022). *How to work with hammers and needles.* Home Press.	Two authors, joined with an ampersand, preceded by a comma.
Histrionik, K. L., Jr., & Stoic, P. L. (2017). *Neurotic behavior* (2nd ed.). Angels Publishing.	Omitted in the text, Jr., is added after the initials in the reference list. A comma precedes the ampersand.
Null, B. D. (2002). *Numbers in civilization* (Rev. ed.). Sappleton.	(Rev. ed.) for revised edition.
Russell, B. (2005). *The analysis of mind.* Dover Publications. (Original work published 1921)	The 2005 publication is a re-issue of the same 1921 publication; the author who cited the book may not have read it in its original print.
Piaget, J., & Inhelder, B. (1969). *The psychology of the child* (H. Weaver, Trans; 2nd ed.). Basic Books. (Original work published in 1966)	A translated book; Trans for translator.
Lahiri, J. (2007). *Interpreter of maladies* (M. Novak, Narr.) [Audiobook]. HighBridge Company.	An audiobook, Narr. for narrator.

Note: The examples are independent of each other (not alphabetized as they should be in a reference list).

Books and Book Chapters

B.4.57b. Authored Books in Reference Lists

Reference Information	Correctly Write the References
Author: K. D. Wong Title: *Bilingual speech-language pathology* Year: 2019 Edition: Second Publisher: Word Publishing Company.	
Authors: S. S. Simms, T. T. Tinns, and K. K. Kimms Title: *Central auditory problems* Year: 2015 Edition: Revised Publisher: Nelson.	
Author: N. C. Gardner and P. T. Smith Title: *Hearing aids of the future* Year: 2017 Publisher: The Future Press.	
Author: American Speech-Language-Hearing Association Title: *Your professional organization* Year: 2015 Publisher: American Speech-Language-Hearing Association	
Author: Jung, C. G Title: Modern man in search of a soul Year: 2017 Translators: W. S. Dell and C. F. Baynes Publisher: Harcourt Brace Original work published in 1933	
Author: Prose, N. (2022). Title: The maid: A novel, an audiobook Year: 2022 Narrator: L. Ambrose Publisher: RB Audiobooks	
Author: J. B. Singleton Title: *Fulfilled single life* Years: 1850, original publication by Companion Press reissued in 2009 by Lonely Press	

B.4.58a. Edited Books and Chapters in Edited Books

- Reference a chapter in an edited book, the entire edited book, or both, depending on what you cited in your text.
- Use the chapter author's name (not the editor's) in alphabetizing the list.
- Unlike the author's initials, place the editor's initials before the surname.
- Enter (Ed.) for one editor or (Eds.) for multiple editors; type (ed.) for the book edition.
- Italicize the book title, not the chapter title.
- Place the chapter pages after the title and within parentheses.
- Copy the entire URL for DOI if available for the book.

Correct	Note
Baker, K. V. (2019). The unconscious. In C. Hart (Ed.), *Unknown states of consciousness* (pp. 305–395). Mystery Publishing House.	In the text, cite the author of the chapter, not the editor (Baker, 2015, not Hart, 2015). The page numbers are for the cited author's chapter only.
Cantun, U. O. (2021). The invisible and the unmeasurable. In K. Panth & C. Hanth (Eds.), *Ghosts within skulls* (2nd ed., pp. 35–95). Ghostly Press.	Chapter cited from the second edition of an edited book. There is no comma after the first editor's name and before the ampersand.
Hunt, C. P., & Holms, G. S. (Eds.). (2001). *Mysteries of mental events*. Invisible Publishers.	This reference is for an entire edited book, not a chapter in it. In the running text, Hunt and Holms (2001); within parentheses, (Hunt & Holms, 2001).
Xong, K. C. (Ed.). (2002). *Split brain is just as good* (2nd ed.). NeuroPress.	Entire edited book is cited in the text. (Ed.) for Editor, (ed.) for edition.
Goldstein, B. (Ed.). (2015–2020). *Speech-language pathology* (Vols. 1–5). Hudson Press.	Reference to a multivolume edited book published over several years. Parenthetical citation in the text: (Goldstein, 2015–2020).
James, J. (Ed.). (2017). *Language disorders.* Retrieved from https://doi.org/10.xxxx	An edited book published only online.
Adams, A. (Ed.). (2015). *Sociology of morality.* https://doi.org/10.xxxx	An online edited publication with only a DOI.

B.4.58b. Edited Books and Chapters in Edited Books

Reference Information	Correctly Write the References
Editors: Johns, L. B., and Bangs, R. K. Book title: *Clinical ethics.* Year: 2017 Publisher: College Press	
Editor: Montu, M. L. Year: 2011 Book: Language therapy in the mind [An online publication with a DOI]	
Author: Jackson, N. O. Chapter title: Speech-language pathologist and the bilingual child Year: 2005 Pages: 135–175 Book title: *Education in the Next Century* Editors: Cantor, A. K., and Bantor, B. L. Publisher: Century Press	
Editor: Lent, B. Years: 2010–2017 Book title: *Speech and Hearing Science* Volumes 1–7 Publisher: Modern Press.	

Conference and Convention Presentations

B.4.59a. Paper and Poster Presentations

- Specify the year and dates
- Specify the town, state, and country

Correct	Note
Peacock, P. L., & Lyon, A. D. (2021, November 18–20). *Communication in the animal kingdom* [Paper presentation]. American Speech-Language-Hearing Association Annual Convention, Washington, DC, United States.	Paper presentation at a convention. Italicize the title of the presentation. "Meeting," "convention," and so forth, should be accurate.
Ram, B. (2017, June 15–16). Case load of school clinicians. In D. Davis (Chair), *Trends in serving school children with communication disorders* [Symposium]. California Speech-Language-Hearing Association 10th Regional Symposium, Fresno, CA, United States.	A paper presentation at a symposium.
Hernandez, K. S. (2022, April 28–30). *Clinician's ethical dilemmas* [Poster presentation]. 2022 Speech-Language Pathology Conference of Speech-Language and Audiology of Canada, Vancouver, BC, Canada.	A poster presentation at a convention.

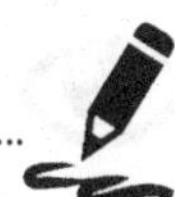

Conference and Convention Presentations

B.4.59b. Paper and Poster Presentations

Reference Information	Correctly Write the References
Author: B. J. Beans Paper presentation: A new method of language sampling Presented at: National Convention of the American Speech-Language-Hearing Association Date: 2018, November 20-22 City: Atlanta, GA, United States	
Author: Ahlander, E. Date: 2016, September 16-17. *Early treatment for stuttering.* Chair: L. Johns. Presented at: Symposium of the Central California Special Education Conference, Clovis Unified School District, Clovis, CA, United States.	
Author: S. Hilton Date: 2020, April 15-18 Poster title: Toddlers are scholars Presented at: Annual Conference of International Child Language Society Place: Sydney, New South Wales, Australia	

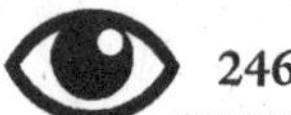

Unpublished Articles, Dissertations, and Theses

B.4.60a. Unpublished Articles, Theses, or Dissertations

Correct	Note
Dimm, B. J. (2020). *Why some articles do not get published* [Unpublished manuscript].	Titles of unpublished works are italicized, while those of published ones are not.
Epson, H. P. (2011). *Levels of aspiration and academic performance* [Unpublished manuscript]. Department of Psychology, University of California, Los Angeles.	An unpublished manuscript obtained from a university department.
Minderson, H. P. (2022). *Do not confuse the brain for the mind* [Manuscript submitted for publication].	A manuscript in the process of being published.
Smiley, S. S. (2017). *Relationship between toilet training and frequency of smiling in high school classrooms* [Unpublished master's thesis]. Sharp College of Education.	Note the brackets: [Unpublished doctoral dissertation] and [Unpublished master's thesis]
Zinson, D. C. (2002). *Fathers' role in children's language learning* [Unpublished doctoral dissertation]. University of Toronto.	
Brightly, B. B. (2014). *Relation between hair color and academic learning*. Retrieved from https://xxxxxxx	If retrieved from an institutional database (such as a university), copy the full URL.

B.4.61a. Theses and Dissertations Published in a Database or Available Online

- Note that dissertations and theses may be available on ProQuest Dissertations and Theses Global.

Correct	Note
Allen, T. H. (2013). *The role of the unconscious in language treatment* [Doctoral dissertation, Unaware University]. ProQuest Dissertations and Theses Global.	Published on the database and accessed online.
Gardner, G. N. (2010). *Horticultural concepts in explaining human behavior* [Master's thesis, Smith College]. Smith College Digital Archive. https://xxxx	Give the institution's full URL.

Unpublished Articles, Dissertations, and Theses

B.4.60b. Unpublished Articles, Theses, or Dissertations

Reference Information	Correctly Write the References
Author: Henkly, T. K. Year, 2015 Unpublished article: How to get published in speech and hearing.	
Author: Carter, J. J. Year, 2012 Unpublished article: Peace on earth. Obtained from: Emory University	
Author: Gyon, G. V. Year, 2010 Unpublished Master's thesis: Evaluation of an early language intervention package. Downstate University	
Author: Meyersson, M. Year, 2022 Unpublished doctoral dissertation: *Mothers' role in her child's cognitive development.* University of London	

B.4.61b. Theses and Dissertations Published in a Database or Available Online

Reference Information	Correctly Write the References
Author: Borgen, T. H. Year 2016 Title: What is in the mind? Searchlight University Doctoral dissertation available on ProQuest Dissertations and Theses Global.	
Author: Branch, L. L. Year, 2013 Title: A plant grows into a tree. Master's theses obtained from the Midstate University archive	

B.4.62 Guidelines on Using Electronic Sources in Scientific Writing

- As noted previously, scientific and scholarly writers cite most of their sources published in peer-reviewed academic journals, published books, and book chapters in edited books. Since the evolution of the internet into a depository of knowledge, however, writers need to cite not only the printed articles and books but also those published online. Many scholarly journals are now published only online, with no print versions. Government departments and agencies and professional organizations publish many valuable pieces of knowledge, guidelines, and summary of scientific information on their websites. These are often expert-reviewed and generally acceptable given the state of research and knowledge.
- Many other sources on the internet, however, including social media and web blogs, offer information that varies in reliability and validity. Social media and blogs may present information that is distorted, highly biased, politically motivated, outright wrong, and purposefully designed to mislead people. Sources and sites may contain opinions and advice without expert evaluations. Therefore, careful, scholarly, scientific, and professional writers should critically evaluate the source to be used in their writing by doing the following:
- *Ascertain who maintains the website.* Is the webpage maintained by a scientific, professional, or governmental agency or organization? Is it owned by an individual? Is it owned by a commercial establishment? Generally speaking, sites owned and managed by scientific, professional, and governmental organizations offer more objective and research-based information than a business that sells products or blogs on which individuals post their opinions. The reader may trust a webpage maintained by an organization whose members are specialists in the topic of interest more than sites that are maintained by novice individuals. For instance, on matters of speech, language, and hearing, http://www.asha.org will be a trustworthy site. On general and specific health matters, the various sites of the National Institutes of Health will be trustworthy. Nonetheless, individuals should critically evaluate what they read on any website.
    - *Find out if it is an advocacy group's site.* If so, consider the information offered as the viewpoints of the host group.
    - *Check whether there are other sources on the internet or in the print media that will help verify the authenticity and validity of claims made.* The site should refer the reader to other sites or sources that will support the information offered. If not, be skeptical. Typically, good documents on the internet have references to reputable sources, such as peer-reviewed journal articles.
    - *Be critical of any extreme or exaggerated claims or statements.* Such statements may not be based on sound research and may not present information from an objective standpoint.
- *Find out if there are sponsors.* If the information on the webpage is filled with advertisers, links, and lures to commercial sites, the information offered should be evaluated in light of such efforts to sell products.
- *Evaluate the information offered on the website for its authorship, reliability, and accuracy.* Who wrote the article on the webpage? Is the author an expert? Is the information based on evidence or scientific research? Is the information offered reviewed by experts? Does the site reference articles published in peer-reviewed journals? Is the information cited a valid representation of articles cited in the journals? Answering the last question is critical because a site may cite references from reputable journals but misrepresent what the articles say.
    - *Find out whether readers edit the information offered on the site.* Although this is not bad in itself, a careful writer would be on alert: The information offered on a site that allows anyone to edit, delete, or add information (e.g., *Wiki* sites) may be considered opinions of people, which may or may not be factual.
    - *Check the currency of information.* The date of posting or updating is important to ascertain. On some of the webpages, decade-old information may be touted.

   - *Always be skeptical of strictly political and personal views expressed on social media.* Do not cite them as valid information, especially on larger socioeconomic and political problems or issues. Cite them only when such matters are themselves the subject of research or an essay.
- On citing information obtained through the internet, the seventh edition of the APA *Manual* (2020) gives more detailed guidelines than given in this book. For a variety of internet source citations, the reader is referred to the *Manual.*
- In citing electronic sources,
   - Follow a general rule of citing the print version whenever available and add electronic retrieval information when that has been supplied as well. Adding DOI and Retrieved from http://www. (ending in the exact URL) will be sufficient in most cases.
   - Follow the reference and citation guidelines that are often found at the right side or at the end of scholarly publications found on materials available online. For example, when you print a document from the website of the American Speech-Language-Hearing Association (ASHA), you may find directions on referencing it at the end of the document. For example, at the end of the document, *Code of ethics*, you find the following:

     Reference this material as: American Speech-Language-Hearing Association. (2016). *Code of ethics* [Ethics]. Available from http://www.asha.org/policy/
   - Shift the elements of the online reference to suit the preferred style (e.g., the APA style); downloaded articles may not follow the APA style.
   - Generally, include the elements you normally would for a print document; however, it is usually not available and is not necessary to specify the geographic location of the webpage publication.
   - Specify the author's name (if available) and the document name or title, not just the home page from which the information was drawn.
   - Give the date of document publication; if unavailable, give the date of retrieval (e.g., Retrieved December 15, 2022). The retrieval date is especially important for documents that change over time because of periodic updates or likely deletion in due course. For example, updates like the following are likely to be modified, edited, or even deleted:

     American Speech-Language Hearing Association. (January 14, 2922). Coronavirus COVID/ updates. Retrieved January 26, 2022, from https://www.asha.org/about/coronavirus-updates/
   - There is no need to specify the retrieval date for books, printed journal articles, and such other materials with a publication date.
   - Give the address, which is the URL; URLs begin with https://www (see the next bullet). Check all the URLs cited in your paper during proofreading (your last chance to make corrections) to make sure that the listed URLs are all active; make necessary corrections.
   - Give the home page URL for online dictionaries and encyclopedias; if the work is permanently archived, a retrieval date is unnecessary. For example:

     Merriam Webster. (n.d.). Words we're watching: Singular 'they': Though singular 'they' is old, 'they' as a nonbinary pronoun is new—And useful. https://www.merriam-webster.com/words-at-play/singular-nonbinary-they

     Graham, G. (2019). Behaviorism. In E. N. Zalta (Ed.), *The Stanford encyclopedia of philosophy* (Spring 2019 ed.). https://plato.stanford.edu/archives/spr2019/entries/behaviorism/
   - Do not add a period at the end of the URL, if there is no period in the address, data path, or directory; do not add any punctuation marks that are not in the original.
   - Use lowercase letters, even for the initial letter of words that start a sentence, if the address, data path, or directory is written that way.

- Cite the source you consulted even though that source may also be available in another form; for instance, if you consulted a printed journal article, cite the printed journal, not its online version, which may also be available.
- Do not include the name of the database in your reference (e.g., it is not necessary to include PubMed or PsycINFO in the reference list).
- Note that *http* and *https* both stand for *hypertext transfer protocol*, a file transfer mechanism recognized by most internet browsers. Of the two, https is secured (encrypted), and http is not. Both are followed by a colon and two forward slashes: http://; https://).
- Include the Digital Object Identifier (DOI) number if one is shown on the journal article you accessed on a database such as ScienceDirect or PubMed. Because the URLs may be changed, moved, or deleted, readers may be unable to find the original source of the article you cite in your work. However, DOIs are relatively stable.
- DOI numbers are usually on the abstract page or the first page of the full text. The DOI is usually a long string of numbers, so to avoid errors, copy it and paste it into your reference list.

Note that a typical URL has the following elements:

- protocol (standard: http://; secured: https://)
- host name, which is often an organization's home page that is generally but not always preceded by http://www. (e.g., http://www.asha.org/ or http://journals.apa.org)
- path to document (e.g., convention02/registration.html)
- single forward slashes separating certain elements in the URL; an example of a full URL is as follows: https://www.asha.org/certification/2020-slp-certification-standards/ (The document is about the speech-language pathology certification standards of the American Speech-Language-Hearing Association.)

Note also that the path name

- is the most case-sensitive of all other elements in the address
- should be reproduced exactly as it appears (including uppercase and lowercase letters and punctuation, if any); it is best to copy and paste
- should not be broken with a hyphen; if you need to break a URL in a typed line, do so after a period or a slash.

B.4.63. Examples of Electronic Sources in the Reference List

Advance Online Publication

Effoe, C. C., Shetty, V., & Shetty, A. K. (2016). Knowledge and attitudes towards human papillomavirus (HPV) among academic and community physicians in Mangalore, India. *Journal of Cancer Education*. Advance online publication. https://doi.org/10.1007/s13187-016-0999-0

Greenwell, T., & Walsh, B. (2021). Evidence-based practice in speech-language pathology: Where are we now? *American Journal of Speech-Language Pathology.* Advance online publication. PubMed ID: 33476190.

ASHA website

American Speech-Language-Hearing Association. (n.d.). *Frequently asked questions: Obtaining reinforcement for stuttering treatment.* https://www.asha.org/practice/reimbursement/private-plans/reimb_stutter_trtmnt/

Facebook page

Little River Canyon National Preserve. (n.d.). *Home* [Facebook page]. Facebook. Retrieved January 12, 2020, from https://www.facebook.com/lirinps/

Journal Article With an Article Number

Jerrentrup, A., Mueller, T., Glowalla, U., Herder, M., Henrichs, N., Neubauer, A., & Schaefer, J. R. (2018). Teaching medicine with the help of "Dr. House." *PLOS ONE, 13*(3), Article e0193972. https://doi.org/10.1371/journal.pone.0193972

Online Publication

U.S. Department of Health and Human Services, National Institutes of Health, National Institute of Mental Health. (2015). NIMH Strategic Plan for Research (NIH Publication No. 02-2650). Retrieved from http://www.nimh.nih.gov/about/strategic-planning-reports/index.shtml

Press Release

National Institute of Mental Health. (2015, March 26). *HIV can spread early, evolve in patients' brains* [Press release]. http://www.nimh.nih.gov/news/science-news/2015/hiv-can-spread-early-evolve-in-patients-brains.shtml

Reference Work Online

Merriam-Webster Dictionary. (n.d.). *Singular nonbinary 'They': Is it 'they are' or 'they' is?* https://www.merriam-webster.com/words-at-play/singular-nonbinary-they-is-or-they-are

Smedly, A. (n.d.). Racism. In *Encyclopedia Britannica.* https://www.britannica.com/topic/racism

Social Media YouTube Posting by a Government Agency

National Institute of Mental Health. (2015, April 14). *"Follow That Cell" prize winners* [Video]. YouTube. https://www.youtube.com/watch?v=lwvsvIPZLUI

Webpage

National Institute of Mental Health. (2013). *Eating disorders.* http://www.nimh.nih.gov/health/topics/eating-disorders/index.shtml

Note to Students Working on Theses or Dissertations

- The graduate schools of most universities and the specific department have a set of guidelines on the preparation of theses and dissertations. The university and the departmental guidelines that generally accept the APA style may have special instructions that deviate in certain respects from the APA style. Therefore, students should follow the guidelines of their department and the graduate school.

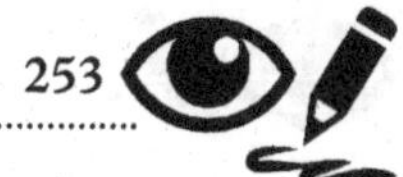

B.5. Writing Sections of Research Papers and Proposals

B.5.1. General Guidelines on Completed and Proposed Empirical Studies

Completed research and a research proposal are different in their content. Generally, the two types of writing follow the same format, including such major headings as Abstract, Method, Results, Discussion, and References. Various subheadings also may be similar if not the same.

Students initially write a thesis or dissertation *proposal* and submit it to a university committee for approval. Upon completion of research, students write a thesis or a dissertation and submit it to their committees. Eventually, theses and dissertations may be written as articles for publication.

Generally, sections of a research proposal are written in the future tense, whereas most sections of a completed study are written in the past tense. There are variations in specific journal styles on these matters. Therefore, authors should read a few sample articles from the journal to which they plan to submit the paper for possible publication and prepare the manuscript according to the guidelines given in the journal.

B.5.2. Sections of a Research Paper

Printed Notes	Class Notes

Abstract

An abstract is a brief description of the problems, the methods, the procedures, and the results of a scientific study in direct, precise, and nonevaluative language. It gives a summary of the article and helps attract the reader to the entire article. Print your abstract on a separate page. In printed journals, abstracts are placed just before the introductory section begins.

The *Publication Manual of the American Psychological Association* (7th ed., 2020; APA *Manual*) restricts an abstract to 250 words. Consult the guidelines of the specific journal that may have a different limit. Use your computer's word processor to automatically count the total number of words, characters, and spaces in the abstract (or any highlighted section of the paper). Write in active voice to use fewer words. Write your own abstracts of a few journal articles you read to practice the art of writing precise and brief abstracts. Reading a few abstracts to learn how they are written also will help. Revise if your abstract sounds vague and exceeds the word limit.

Printed Notes	Class Notes

There are two types of abstracts across different journals. Some abstracts are in a single paragraph with no headings. Other abstracts, like those found in the journals of the American Speech-Language-Hearing Association, use a structure that includes the headings: Purpose, Method, Results, Conclusions, each written in a separate paragraph. Follow your target journal guideline.

At the end of *Conclusions*, list any **supplementary materials** you have assembled for the paper. Placed online, these include video or audio clips, animation, detailed treatment procedures, extensive tables, color figures, and so forth. An example from ASHA's *Language, Speech, and Hearing Services in Schools* looks like this:

Supplemental Material: https://doi.org/10.23641/asha.17003980

If the journal requires it, write a few important terms defined and described in your paper. Place them under a heading *Key Words* (in italics), just below the abstract, indented 0.5 in. like a regular paragraph. All key words, except for proper nouns, should be in lowercase letters. Key words may be used to index the terms in the article. ASHA journals do not list key words.

Introduction

Begin the text of the paper with an untitled introductory section. Do not type "Introduction," although you might use topical headings within the introduction. In this section, introduce (a) the general area of investigation; (b) the general findings of past investigations; (c) the specific topic of the current investigation; (d) a review of selected studies that have dealt with the topic in the past; (e) the methods, results, conclusions, methodological problems, and limitations of the past studies; (f) the questions that remain to be answered; (g) the significance of the current investigation; and (h) the specific problem or research questions investigated in the present study.

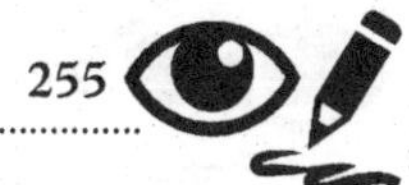

Printed Notes	Class Notes

Your introduction should move from the general topic of investigation to the particular research question you investigated. Critically review previous studies to set the stage for your investigation and to point out gaps in knowledge. Write a fair, objective, and direct review. Make it clear to the reader the need for the study and the reasoning behind it. Relate your study to past research, and point out the innovative methods you have designed.

Toward the end of the introduction, state the research question. If you prefer, state your hypotheses. Write the research questions and hypotheses in direct, clear, and terse language. A good introduction gives sufficient background to the study and justifies its execution. By the end of this section, the reader should gain a clear understanding of the context of your study and why you did it.

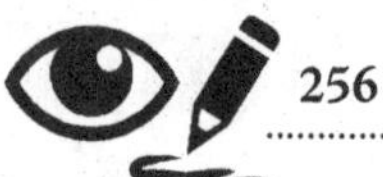

Printed Notes	Class Notes

Method

In the second major section, describe the method in detail to (a) give sufficient information on the methods and procedures of your study so the reader may judge their appropriateness to answer the research questions and (b) permit direct and systematic replications of the study.

The method section consists of at least three subsections: (a) the participants, (b) the apparatus or materials, and (c) the procedure. Use additional subsections (and subheadings), such as Randomization, Baselines, Experiment 1, and Experiment 2, as may be found necessary.

Do not confuse the method with procedures. A broader term than *procedures*, Method is a Level 1 heading, and *Procedures* is a Level 2 heading.

Participants

Describe the relevant characteristics of the participants, including gender, gender identity, age, education, cultural background, occupation, family background, health, geographic location, and communicative behaviors. Specify the number of participants and how you selected them.

In clinical studies, describe the participants' diseases and disorders in both qualitative and quantitative terms. Generally, describe any subject characteristic that may influence the results.

Describe the ethnocultural background of your study participants. Identify an ethnocultural group in the most precise terms possible. For example, instead of describing participants as Asian Americans, specify, for example, that 20 Vietnamese and 20 Japanese American cisgender women participated in the study. Such specificity helps determine the generality of reported findings.

To write about participants of different ethnocultural background and gender identity in an unbiased style, see section B.2. Terms for Writing Without Bias.

Printed Notes	Class Notes

Materials

In this subsection, describe the physical setting of the study and the names and model numbers of equipment used. Simply mention the routine equipment such as furniture but describe in detail any scientific or electronic instrument you used, including the name of the manufacturer and the model number. Describe in sufficient detail the instruments you fabricated.

Summarize the standardized or nonstandardized tests and other assessment or rating procedures. If the apparatus is unusual or rarely used, include photographs, diagrams, or additional descriptions. Some or all of that may be placed online as supplementary materials.

Procedures

Describe in detail how you conducted the study. Specify the experimental design. Describe and justify uncommon design. Describe all stimuli presented to the subjects (including instructions given), how you measured and manipulated the variables, and the temporal sequence of various conditions arranged in the study.

Describe how your experimental and control group participants differed, as well as the procedures for establishing reliability of the data. In reporting clinical treatment studies, describe the treatment procedures and how you implemented them. Specify the methods by which you measured and evaluated the treatment effects.

Other procedural information unique to the study may be included in this section. In making this section complete, follow the rule of providing all information necessary for another investigator to replicate your study.

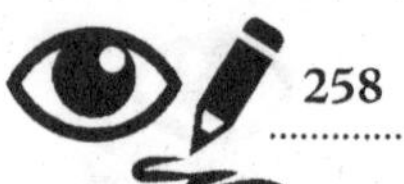

Printed Notes	Class Notes

Results

Open the results section with a brief statement of the problem investigated and the general findings of the study. Following this overview, present the quantitative, qualitative, graphic, and tabular presentations of the findings. Report these findings without evaluations and interpretations.

Use tables and graphs to display data and to supplement, not duplicate, the text. Specify and, when necessary, justify the statistical or other procedures of data analysis.

In organizing the results of a study, consult the APA *Manual* and several exemplary articles published in the professional journal to which you plan to submit the paper for publication.

Discussion

In the discussion section, point out the meaning and significance of the results. Open this section with a brief statement of the problem and the major findings. Discuss the theoretical and applied implications of the findings. Relate the current findings to those of previous investigations.

Finally, point out the study limitations and suggest the need for further research. A discussion is an integrative essay on the topic investigated, but write it in light of the study's data. Answer the research questions posed in the introduction and support or refute any hypotheses presented. Aim for clarity and directness. Avoid excessive speculation on the causes of unexpected data that refute your initial hypotheses.

References

List publications and other sources of information cited in the paper. Prepare an accurate list according to the guidelines given in the journal to which you plan to submit your paper. List all, and only, the sources cited in the paper.

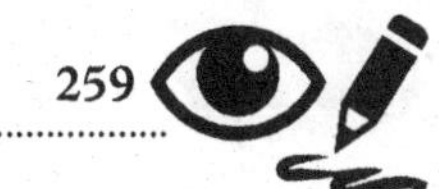

Note to Students on Different Formats of Journal Articles

Besides research papers (empirical reports), scientific and professional journals publish review papers, theoretical papers, tutorials, commentaries on articles published in the journal, opinion pieces, clinical focus, research notes, letters to the editor, and other kinds of papers. Each type of paper has a prescribed format. Consult the journals in your discipline to understand the types and formats of publications.

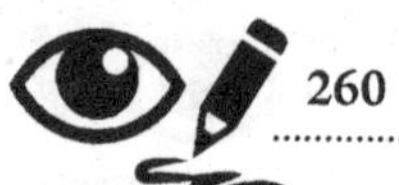

B.6. Manuscript Submission, Revision, and Proofreading

B.6.1. Manuscript Submission for Journal Publication

Printed Notes	Class Notes

Authors may upload their finished research papers to a manuscript submission portal maintained by the journal or an association such as the American Speech-Language-Hearing Association (ASHA). Authors electronically receive reviews of their manuscripts, the copyedited versions, and the page proofs.

Electronic manuscript submission guidelines are becoming more standardized but still vary across journals. Different publishers of journals have different online submission portals. The guidelines vary across journals, disciplines, and organizations and are subject to changes. Therefore, only a general overview of submission procedures for the journals of the American Speech-Language-Hearing Association is provided here. Authors should get specific and detailed guidelines that apply to the journal selected for submission.

ASHA journals are continuously published online. Authors may search and read 60 years of archived articles. ASHAWire is the online site where you can read the articles. Through emails, members receive the *table of contents* of each new issue published online. Members may download the articles, store on their own computers, or print them. Printed paper copies, ePrint of an entire issue, or a particular article may be ordered for a fee.

All ASHA journals use the style of the *Publication Manual of the American Psychological Association* (APA style) and accept papers only through their electronic submission portal. The ASHA Journals Academy (https://academy.pubs.asha.org) offers all the information needed to submit an article for consideration. To submit a paper to one of the ASHA journals, authors should log on to the ASHA website: http://www.asha.org, click on "Publications" for general information, and then select a journal for submission. The selected journal site offers specific guidelines on the kinds of articles that may be submitted, writing and formatting the article, the peer review process, and the steps involved in the production of the article in an issue.

Printed Notes	Class Notes

ASHA uses a portal called the Editorial Manager maintained by the Aries Systems to receive manuscripts, edit them, get them reviewed, communicate the review and revision suggestions to the authors, receive the revised manuscript, and make the final judgment of acceptance or rejection. Revised and accepted articles may be uploaded to ProduXion Manager for publication in the journal. Because these procedures undergo updates and changes, it is the author's responsibility to visit the journal website to find and follow the latest guidelines.

ASHA also maintains journals author services (https://authorservices.pubs.asha.org) that offers help with English editing, plagiarism check, artwork preparation, translation from other languages, research communication, and rapid technical review that helps avoid common reasons for rejection. The author pays for these services.

The editor or the associate editor of journals will send all articles submitted for possible publication to editorial reviewers. The publication of the article is contingent on the reviewers' recommendations. If the article is not acceptable because of faulty procedures, insignificant research questions investigated, and other reasons, the author may receive a rejection letter.

If the article is otherwise acceptable but needs a revision, the editor will summarize the main points of the reviews, add their own comments and suggestions, and ask the author to make the recommended changes. It will be up to the author to accept or reject the suggestions. Although there is no guarantee of final acceptance of the paper, the author who makes the recommended changes and resubmits the paper may improve the chances of getting it published in the journal.

When an article is submitted on the journal's portal, an account for the particular submission is created. The author will access the secured portal with a password for reviews and editor's comments. The author may receive an email alert to check progress on the submission.

B.6.2. Submission for Convention or Conference Presentations

Printed Notes	Class Notes

Most professional organizations, including ASHA and state associations, invite papers to be submitted online for presentations at their annual conventions or other kinds of conferences. Formats for convention and conference presentations vary, depending on the type of presentation (e.g., oral presentations, posters, symposia, workshops, etc.). The format for specific kinds of presentations also varies across organizations.

Online submission guidelines for convention and conference presentations are periodically updated with newer and more user-friendly features. Therefore, presenters should consult the latest guidelines in preparing their oral or poster presentation proposals. Email invitations that organizations send to their members to submit proposals contain links to the site on which the authors may prepare their proposals.

B.6.3. Book and Book Chapter Publications

Printed Notes	Class Notes

Most publishers accept book and book chapters as email attachments. Authors may also use a site where files are shared (e.g., the Dropbox). The author must follow the style manual of the publishing house to which the book manuscript is expected to be submitted. Most publishers expect the manuscript to be prepared in Microsoft Word or Mac Word formats.

Book manuscripts do not strictly conform to the APA style or any other standard style (e.g., the Modern Language Association, American Medical Association, or Chicago styles). Each book publishing company has its own style manual, although many in behavioral sciences (including speech-language pathology) follow the general guidelines of APA or another standard style, particularly in citing authors in the text and creating the reference list. Medically oriented book publishers may follow elements of the American Medical Association's style manual.

Printed Notes	Class Notes

Unlike journal articles, books are designed with a concern for readability, aesthetic appeal, and pedagogical devices that help readers learn the information the books offer. Journal articles are faithful to the selected style. Books, however, may differ in their style. For example, heading styles may be distinctly different in a book that otherwise generally follows the APA style.

The in-house editor of the book publishing company is likely to send the manuscript to selected expert reviewers, similar to those who review journal articles. These reviewers will critically examine the book for its coverage, content, writing style, currency in the discipline, clarity of expression, accuracy of information presented, research base of the claims made, and usefulness to the intended audience. They may have general comments about the writing style and adherence to the selected style (e.g., the APA style), but their main concern is the content and scope of the book.

The manuscript comes back to the author with reviews and suggestions for improvement. The author revises the manuscript in light of the reviews and sends it back to the editor at the publishing house.

B.6.4. Copyediting and Author Revisions

Printed Notes	Class Notes

An in-house or a hire-for-contract *copy editor* will edit the book manuscript in the Word format. Although not a content expert, the copy editor is a master of clear and precise writing style. The copy editor offers suggestions to improve the manuscript's readability, accuracy, consistency, and grammaticality. The copy editor also checks the reference list and alerts the author to discrepancies between the cited and referenced sources. The copy editor ensures strict adherence to the selected style guide and edits the manuscript for stylistic uniformity. They will query the author about errors, oversights, omissions, ambiguities, and confusing sentences and offer suggestions for changes.

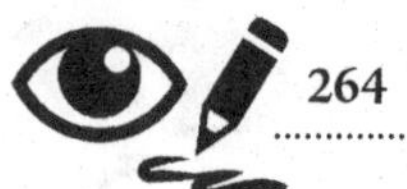

Printed Notes	Class Notes

Because the copyeditor will have turned on the "Track Changes" function under Review in the Word program screen, all changes made will be shown in a different color font. Comments, queries, and revision suggestions may be shown in the right-hand margin.

The copyedited manuscript comes back to the author for a final revision. This is true for both book manuscripts and journal articles. The author also will be expected to turn on the "Track Changes" function in Word so the editor can see the changes made in the document. This is the last opportunity for the author to revise the manuscript.

B.6.5. Proofreading

Printed Notes	Class Notes

The publishing house, upon receiving the final version of the manuscript, will convert the file into a PDF (Portable Document Format) to design the article or book, typeset, and create page proofs. PDF page proofs look like a printed article or book. To accurately proof the pages and respond to any queries, the author should have learned to use the editing features of PDF documents.

In reading the page proofs, authors are allowed to correct only any remaining spelling or factual errors. Rewriting the manuscript is not allowed. Authors who make extensive changes in the proofs may be asked to pay for those changes. Authors electronically send the reviewed page proofs back to the publisher. After a final round of corrections, the PDF file is sent to the printer for printing and binding. In due course, authors will see their work in print.

PART C

Professional Writing

C.1. Introduction to Professional Writing

Professional writing includes writing diagnostic or assessment reports, treatment plans, progress reports, and professional correspondence. As there is no standard accepted by all clinics, the headings and the formats of these reports vary. Furthermore, *clinical reports need not follow all aspects of the style of the Publication Manual of the American Psychological Association (APA style)*, which is most relevant to scientific writing. Unlike research articles, clinical reports may use different margins, paragraph styles, indentations, phrases (incomplete sentences), one-sentence paragraphs, and bulleted lists. However, like other kinds of writing, professional writing also should be clear, brief, objective, and nonbiased.

The following pages offer examples of various clinical reports. Student clinicians, clinical supervisors, or instructors may use these as examples only; they are not meant to be prescriptive. Nonetheless, it is better for the beginning student to master a format than to enter clinical practicum with no such format. Experienced clinicians will have learned to vary the style to suit their employment setting and audience.

Clinicians in public schools, medical settings, and university clinics write vastly different kinds of reports. Reports vary in their formats and details. Assessment reports may be a single page or several pages. Some contain connected prose; others contain only symbols, abbreviations, phrases, and brief observations. Generally, reports written in medical settings are briefer than those written in university speech and hearing clinics. Therefore, some student clinicians in university clinics ask why they are expected to write detailed reports that are uncommon in the "real world."

There are at least two good reasons for teaching student clinicians how to write reports with complete sentences and connected prose. First, even settings that routinely require brief reports with notes and notations on occasion require detailed, formal reports with extensive supportive evidence. When treatment has to be justified to a third party who pays for services or when a report comprehensible to other professionals has to be written, the clinician has to use a more narrative, cogent, and well-organized style. Second, the one who knows how to write a detailed report should have very little trouble writing brief reports. But the clinician who has learned only a brief and disconnected style will have great difficulty in writing elaborate, well-reasoned, well-organized narrative reports when needed.

Student clinicians should study the examples carefully and compare them with those written in their clinic. A simple rule of clinical practicum is to follow the guidelines of the setting in which that experience is offered. Therefore, it is the student clinicians' responsibility to find out what is acceptable in their setting.

C.2. Elements of Diagnostic Reports

Diagnostic reports are also known as *assessment reports* and *evaluation reports*. Those three terms may be used interchangeably. Choose the term that is used in your setting.

Common Elements of a Diagnostic Report

Although the formats vary, all diagnostic reports contain the following kinds of information:

- history of the client, the family, and the disorder
- relevant medical history
- interview of the family, the client, or both
- orofacial examination
- hearing screening
- speech and language samples
- disorder-specific assessment, including standardized and client-specific assessment procedures
- diagnostic summary
- recommendations

Unique Elements Depending on the Age of the Client

Children

Generally, assessment of children and adolescents requires more detailed information on the following:

- medical history of pregnancy and birth
- childhood diseases including middle ear infections
- early and subsequent speech, motor, and general behavioral development
- family, social, and educational history
- effects of the communication disorder on the child's education and socialization

Adults

- more recent medical history
- living arrangements, family, and social history
- educational and occupational history
- effects of the communication disorder on the adult's personal, social, and work life

Older Individuals

- all information included for adults
- health and diseases associated with older age, especially neurologic disorders (stroke, tumors), potential physical and cognitive decline, social isolation, family support or its absence, extended care needs, financial needs, independent living skills, and so forth

On the following pages, examples of diagnostic reports are presented. Note the following:

- The various headings and subheadings may vary across clinics and clinicians.
- Most clinicians include information of the kind the headings suggest.
- All headings and subheadings are not needed for all clients.

C.3. Diagnostic Reports

Note to Student Clinicians

On the following pages, samples of diagnostic (assessment) reports are presented. Study them for the general content and format of diagnostic reports. Compare the samples with the format used in your clinic. Take note of variations in headings and their styles used in your clinic. Consult with your clinic director or clinical supervisor to select an approved format and acceptable variations, if any.

C.3.1. Diagnostic Report: *Speech Sound Disorder*

University Speech and Hearing Clinic
Midstate University
Middletown, Montana

Diagnostic Report

Client: Pennifer Forbes	Date of Birth: xx-xx-xxxx
Address:	Clinic File Number: 9-Qr101
City: Middletown, Montana	Date of Report: xx-xx-xxxx
Telephone Number:	Diagnosis: Phonological Disorder
Referred By: Jane Pendelton, MD	Clinician: Missouline Montoya

Background and Reasons for Referral

Pennifer Forbes, a 5-year, 4-month-old female, was seen on February x, xxxx, for an evaluation at the Speech and Hearing Clinic at the Midstate University, Middletown, Montana. Dr. Pendelton, a pediatrician, referred her to the clinic because of her articulation problems. Pennifer was accompanied to the clinic by her mother, Mrs. Jane Forbes, who served as the informant.

History

Mrs. Forbes reported that Pennifer's speech is difficult to understand. She said that her daughter leaves out sounds in her speech resulting in such words as "nake" for "snake." Pennifer also substitutes one sound for another. The mother reported that Pennifer says, "tat" for "cat." Pennifer has previously received speech therapy at Big Sky Speech and Hearing Center for remediation of her speech sound disorder. The 3-month treatment she received resulted in some improvement, but Pennifer's speech problems are still significant.

Pennifer's birth and developmental history is not remarkable. Her motor and speech development was typical, as judged by Mrs. Forbes. Pennifer has enjoyed good health with no diseases of significance.

Family, Social, and Educational History

Pennifer is the second of three children. Mrs. Forbes did not report a family history of communication problems. Mrs. Forbes, a high school graduate, manages a restaurant. Mr. Forbes, who has a 10th-grade education, is a maintenance man with the local school district.

Pennifer attends a kindergarten school and is reportedly doing well. However, other students and the teacher have complained about her unintelligible speech.

Assessment Information

Orofacial Examination

An orofacial examination was performed to assess the function and integrity of the oral and facial structures. Pennifer's lips and hard palate appeared symmetrical at rest. She was able to perform a variety of labial and lingual tasks. The anterior and posterior faucial pillars were within normal limits. Vertical movement of the pharyngeal wall was observed upon the phonation of /a/.

Hearing Screening

Using a Maico Pilot Test Audiometer, the clinician screened Pennifer's hearing at 25 dB hearing level (HL) for 500, 1000, 2000, and 4000 Hz. At all frequencies, Pennifer passed the screening bilaterally.

Speech Sound Production and Speech Intelligibility

To assess Pennifer's speech sound production, a conversational speech sample was recorded. In addition, the Goldman–Fristoe Test of Articulation (GFTA) was administered to assess speech sounds in fixed positions. An analysis of the speech sample and Pennifer's performance on the GFTA revealed the following errors:

	Initial	Medial	Final
Substitutions	/s/ for /k/; /d/ for /g/; /t/ for /s/; /w/ for /r/; /b/ for /f/; /t/ for /ʧ/; /t/ for /ʃ/; /j/ for /z/; /b/ for /bl/; /b/ for /br/; /d/ for /dr/; /bl/ for /fl/; /t/ for /kl/; /l/ for /sl/; /d/ for /st/	/l/ for /t/; /t/ for /ʃ/; /b/ for /v/; /d/ for /g/; /b/ for /f/; /t/ for /ʧ/	/k/ for /t/; /p/ for /b/
Omissions		/k/ and /θ/	/g/, /k/, /d/, /f/, /s/, /t/, /ʃ/, /ʧ/, /θ/, /l/, /d/, /z/, /p/
Distortions		/z/	

The Khan–Lewis Phonological Analysis was administered to assess Pennifer's phonological error patterns. Pennifer's overall score of 32 on the test was calculated into an age equivalency of 2 years, 9 months. The analysis revealed the following phonological patterns:

- deletion of final consonants
- palatal fronting
- velar fronting
- stridency deletion
- stopping of affricates and fricatives
- cluster simplification
- final devoicing
- liquid simplification

Because of numerous speech sound errors, only 33% of Pennifer's utterances without context were intelligible. In addition, most of her misarticulations were not stimulable. Pennifer correctly imitated only /k/, /g/, /s/, and /f/. However, a diadochokinetic test showed rates within normal limits.

Language Production and Comprehension

Pennifer's conversational speech during the interview and assessment showed normal language structure and use except for several missing grammatical morphemes. Possibly, some missing speech sounds coincide with missing grammatical morphemes. The mean length of utterance (MLU) of her speech sample was 5.4 morphemes, which is within normal limits for her age.

Voice and Fluency

Though difficult to understand, Pennifer's speech had normal rhythm. Because the dysfluency frequency was within the normal range, no further analysis of fluency was made. In addition, Pennifer's voice was judged to be within normal limits.

Diagnostic Summary

Pennifer Forbes exhibited a severe speech sound disorder characterized by multiple errors and limited speech intelligibility. Because of the various speech sound error patterns found in her speech, diagnosis of a phonological disorder is justified. Untreated, her speech sound disorder is likely to have negative social and educational consequences. Because Pennifer was stimulable for some of the consonants, the prognosis with treatment for improved speech intelligibility is good.

Recommendations

It is recommended that Pennifer receive treatment for her phonological disorder. As her production of speech sound accuracy and intelligibility improve, Pennifer's language may be further evaluated to see if morphological features emerge. If they do not, language treatment may be offered.

Submitted By ______________________________

Missouline Montoya, BA
Student Clinician

Parent's Signature ______________________________

Jane Forbes, Mother

Approved By ______________________________

Akbar Jamal, MA, CCC-SLP
Speech-Language Pathologist
Clinical Supervisor

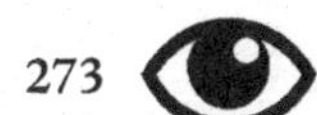

C.3.2. Diagnostic Report: *Voice Disorder*

Balmtown University Speech and Hearing Clinic
Balmtown, New York

Diagnostic Report

Name: Valine Wrenn

Date of Birth: xx-xx-xxxx

Age: 25 years

Address:

City:

Telephone:

Date of Examination: xx-xx-xxxx

Clinical Classification: Voice Disorder

Clinic File No: 08a-7314

Referred By: Dr. Hanna Eismer

Examiner: Janina Presham

Informant: Self

Background and Presenting Complaints

Valine Wrenn, a 25-year-old female, was seen for a speech and language evaluation at the Balmtown University Speech and Hearing Clinic on April xx, xxxx. She was referred to the clinic by her otolaryngologist, Dr. Eismer. Her presenting complaints were difficulty speaking loudly and sustaining voice for longer periods of speaking. She also noted a "lack of excitement" in her voice and difficulty producing sounds at the ends of sentences caused by a low pitch. Valine came to the clinic by herself and provided all the information.

History

Early History

Valine reported that her voice always sounded "funny" since early childhood. During her high school years, she became aware of a low pitch and monotone quality when she listened to her own voice recordings. Valine did not recall previous consultations or treatment for her voice problem. She thought that her developmental history was unremarkable.

Medical History

On March xx, xxxx, Valine received a medical evaluation by Dr. Hanna Eismer, an otolaryngologist. Dr. Eismer reported Valine as having normal external auditory canals and tympanic membranes. The nose and oral cavities were clear. A fiberoptic endoscope was used to examine Valine's larynx. Vocal fold structure and motion were reported to be normal. There was no evidence of vocal nodules or lesions. The vocal folds were described as being minimally erythematous (redness of tissue) and slightly swollen on the free edge.

Valine is allergic to such substances as molds, trees, and grasses. When she is close to one of them, phlegm in the throat and postnasal drip tend to increase. Valine recently began using Beconase (an inhalant) to relieve the allergies. Valine typically experiences excessive colds resulting in phlegm and postnasal drip approximately once a month beginning in October or November, and lasting about a week. Valine thought that her colds were caused by stress and emotional problems. She temporarily discontinued the use of the Beconase while using Afrin and Neo-Synephrine for the colds. Excessive phlegm resulted in frequent coughing and throat clearing.

Family, Social, and Educational History

Valine is a student at Balmtown University, Balmtown, New York, majoring in speech communication. She is divorced and lives with her 3-year-old daughter, Haline. Either the television or the radio is on in Valine's apartment for the majority of the time she is at home. While speaking to her daughter, Valine rarely shouts or yells through the apartment. Instead, she goes into the room where her daughter is. Valine noted that she frequently sings for personal pleasure. She sings in numerous and varied settings, including at home, in the car, and on campus. She has between two to five telephone conversations per day, ranging from 2 to 30 minutes in length. Valine does not habitually drink coffee, tea, soft drinks, or alcoholic beverages. She does drink at least two glasses of low-fat milk every day. Valine mentioned that friends easily identify her voice and describe it as being "low and sexy." Valine typically experiences a feeling of tightness in the throat when nervous, as well as a higher pitch, lower intensity, and difficulty projecting her voice.

Assessment Information

Orofacial Examination

An orofacial examination was conducted to assess the integrity of oral and facial structures. Valine's facial features appeared symmetrical, with lingual and labial mobility adequate for speech. However, restricted oral mobility was noted during speech. Velopharyngeal closure was acoustically deemed adequate during repeated productions of /a/. Diadochokinetic rates were within normal limits.

Hearing Screening

Using a Grason Stadler GS18 Audiometer, the clinician screened Valine's hearing at 25 dB HL for 500, 1000, 2000, and 4000 Hz. At all frequencies, Valine passed the screening bilaterally.

Speech Sound Production and Comprehension

Valine's speech production and comprehension were informally assessed. Her conversational speech and her interaction during the interview did not reveal speech sound errors or comprehension problems. Therefore, these aspects of her communicative behaviors were judged to be within normal variations.

Language and Fluency

Valine's language and fluency were assessed informally. Her conversational speech during the assessment period did not suggest problems of language structure or use. Her fluency and rates of dysfluencies were judged to be within normal variations.

Voice

Valine's fundamental frequency ranged between 150 Hz and 200 Hz on the fundamental frequency indicator. This pitch was determined to be low for Valine's gender and stature. During the interview, frequent glottal fry and hoarseness of voice were observed. A later analysis of the recorded speech sample revealed that glottal fry and hoarseness were more likely to occur on downward inflections of most utterances. On approximately 60% of her utterances, either glottal fry, hoarseness, or both were observed. However, Valine's breath support appeared adequate for speech.

 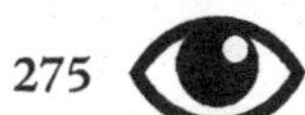

Diagnostic Summary

Valine Wrenn's history suggests vocally abusive behaviors. She uses a habitual pitch that is too low for her. This may have resulted in excessive glottal fry. Her low vocal focus may have adversely affected the extent to which she could project her voice.

Recommendations

It was recommended that Valine Wrenn receive voice therapy. Valine was found to be stimulable for higher pitch levels. Therefore, prognosis for improved pitch level under treatment was judged to be good. Specific recommendations for treatment include the following:

1. Eliminate glottal fry by raising Valine's habitual pitch to a more optimal level during spontaneous conversational speech produced in nonclinical settings.
2. Decrease such abusive vocal behaviors as ineffective management of colds and allergies, improper fluid intake, and singing and speaking in noisy situations.

Submitted By ______________________________

Janina Presham, BA
Student Clinician

Client's Signature ______________________________

Valine Wrenn

Approved By ______________________________

Dambly Doumbleson, MA, CCC-SLP
Clinical Supervisor
Speech-Language Pathologist

C.3.3. Diagnostic Report: *Aphasia and Apraxia of Speech*

University Speech and Hearing Clinic
Tinkyville, Tennessee

Diagnostic Report

Name: Lynn M. Zoolanfoos	Date of Birth: xx-xx-xxxx
Address:	Clinic File Number: 910019
City:	Diagnosis: Aphasia and Apraxia
Telephone Number:	Date of Report: xx-xx-xxxx
Clinician: Maxine Traoumer	Supervisor: Galaxy Galvestrouton, MA, CCC-SLP
Referred By: Dr. Mendelsohn	Assessment Date: xx-xx-xx

Background and Reasons for Referral

Lynn Zoolanfoos, a 44-year-old female, was referred to the Speech and Hearing Clinic at the Tinkyville State University, Tinkyville, Tennessee. Her physician, Dr. Muskwhiter Mendelsohn, referred her for a speech-language evaluation following a stroke.

Lynn's speech and language were evaluated in two sessions. She was seen on September xx, xxxx, and October xx, xxxx. Lynn was unaccompanied to the diagnostic sessions. She suffered an initial stroke in July xxxx. On September xx, xxxx, she experienced a second stroke that resulted in right hemiplegia, expressive and receptive aphasia, and apraxia of speech.

History

Medical History

Lynn has a history of heart problems. She resides with her mother, Gladys Miller, who experiences severe emphysema and is on continuous oxygen. Lynn and her mother have a home care aide who comes into the home 6 hours a day.

Lynn reported she wears braces on her right leg and right hand and uses a cane to assist with walking. Lynn enjoys activities such as bowling and watching television. She now wants to improve her writing skills.

Previous Speech and Language Services

For the past 6 months, Lynn has received speech and language services at the Community Hospital Speech and Hearing Department. Previous treatment targets include the production of two- to four-word phrases, correct production of initial and final consonants in single words, auditory comprehension of two- and three-step directions and two- and three-element questions, and reading comprehension of three- to six-word sentences.

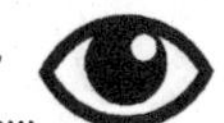

Assessment Information

Lynn cooperated during the evaluation and showed excellent motivation for continuing therapy. She was keenly interested in the assessment tasks. She said that she wanted to improve her speech and language skills.

Orofacial Examination

An orofacial examination was performed to evaluate the functional and structural integrity of the oral and facial complex. Facial features including lips at rest were judged symmetrical and normal in appearance and function. The tongue was normal in appearance, but its lateral movements were sluggish. There were groping behaviors while attempting to draw the tip of the tongue along the hard palate. A slight neutroclusion was noted. The hard palate was narrow, with a high arch and a small bony outgrowth along the midline. Pronounced rugae were evident in the premaxillary region. The soft palate was of adequate length and elevated vertically and posteriorly to achieve closure. Velopharyngeal functioning was acoustically judged to be adequate during production of /a/. An assessment of diadochokinetic rates revealed slowness suggesting weakness in circumoral and lingual musculature. The productions also were characterized by substitutions suggesting apraxia of speech.

Voice

Lynn's voice characteristics were subjectively judged based on her conversational speech. Except for a hyponasal resonance, her voice was judged appropriate for her age and gender.

Hearing Screening

Using Earscan 3 ES3S Audiometer, Lyn's hearing was screened bilaterally at 25 dB HL for 500, 1000, 2000, and 4000 Hz. She passed at all frequencies bilaterally.

Speech Production

The Apraxia Battery for Adults was administered to verify the presence of apraxia of speech and provide a rough estimate of the severity of the disorder. Lynn's scores were as follows:

Lynn's scores on the subtests

Subtest I	Diadochokinetic Rate
Pt	13
Tk	10
Ptk	6
Subtest II	Increasing Word Length
1-syllable average	1.8
2-syllable average	1.7
3-syllable average	1.9
Deterioration in Performance Score	0
Subtest III	Limb and Oral Apraxia
Limb Apraxia	34
Oral Apraxia	39

Subtest IV	Latency and Utterance Time for Polysyllabic Words
Latency Time	93 seconds
Utterance Time	2 seconds
Subtest V	Repeated Trials Test
Total Amount of Change	+1
Subtest VI	Inventory of Articulation Characteristics of Apraxia of Speech
Total Yes Items	2

Lynn's performance on the subtests reveals searching behaviors for making gestures and a low score on articulation characteristics of apraxia of speech.

Language Production and Comprehension

A 76-utterance, 157-word language sample was obtained. The mean length for these utterances was 2.19 for words and 2.42 for morphemes. Word-finding difficulties were noted. Automatic speech was evident in some of her replies.

To make an initial assessment of Lynn's aphasia, the first three items of each subtest of the Western Aphasia Battery were administered as a screening test. In the following table, Lynn's scores are listed in the left-hand column. Several subtests were scored beyond the first three items. These scores are listed in the right-hand column. The scores were as follows:

	Lynn's Subscores on First Three Items/Maximum	Lynn's Subscores Beyond the First Three Items/Maximum
Spontaneous Speech		
Information content	6/10	
Fluency	5/10	
Yes/no questions	9/9	36/42
Auditory word recognition	9/27	
Sequential commands	6/6	8/22
Repetition	6/6	60/70
Word fluency	2/20	
Sentence completion	4/6	6/10
Responsive speech	0/6	
Reading	20.5/32	30.5/52
Writing	31.5/100	
Praxis	6/6	27/30
Drawing	3/9	
Calculation	0/4	

Lynn performed well on tasks involving auditory comprehension for yes/no questions, auditory comprehension of one-part sequential commands, verbal repetition of single words and two- to five-word phrases, sentence completion, and reading single words. Errors were noted during tasks involving oral reading of phrases and sentences, spelling, writing (except for writing numbers and her own name and copying printed words), calculation, drawing, responsive speech, word fluency, auditory word recognition, spontaneous speech, and two-part sequential commands. Lynn's performance on the Praxis subtest did not suggest oral or verbal apraxia. An Aphasia Quotient and a Cortical Quotient were unobtainable because of partial presentation of the test.

Diagnostic Summary

Lynn's performance on various assessment tasks suggested a moderate to severe expressive and receptive aphasia with anomia. A mild apraxia of speech was also evident.

Recommendations

Speech and language treatment is recommended for Lynn. With treatment, prognosis for improved communication skills is judged to be good because of the high levels of motivation and cooperation Lynn showed during assessment. Immediate treatment goals recommended for her include the following:

- improved expressive language
- consistent productions of selected functional words and phrases; productions may include a variety of communication modes (gesturing, drawing, speaking, writing) to improve communicative effectiveness
- four- to six-word sentence completion performance with 90% accuracy
- improved receptive language in reading
- correct responses with 90% accuracy to questions about silently read material

Submitted By ______________________________

Maxine Traoumer, BA
Student Clinician

Client's Signature ______________________________

Lynn Zoolanfoos

Approved By ______________________________

Galaxy Galvestrouton, MA, CCC-SLP
Speech-Language Pathologist
Clinical Supervisor

C.3.4. Diagnostic Report: *Stuttering*

University Speech and Hearing Clinic
Freemont University
Valleyville, California

Diagnostic Report

Name: James Foxx

Date of Birth: xx-xx-xxxx

Address:

City:

Telephone Number:

Referred By: Self

Assessment Date: xx-xx-xxxx

File Number: Rs92019

Diagnosis: Stuttering

Date of Report: xx-xx-xxxx

Informant: Self

Clinician: Meena Wong

Background and Presenting Complaint

James Foxx, a 21-year-old male, was seen for a speech and language evaluation at the Freemont University Speech and Hearing Clinic on February x, xxxx. He had applied for services for his stuttering after he read an article in the campus newspaper about the speech and hearing services on campus. James is a student at the university, majoring in computer science.

History

James's parents had told him that his stuttering began when he was about 3 years of age. From the age of 4 through 9 years, James received treatment for his stuttering at J. R. Cronin Elementary School in Dublin, California. At age 7 years, he also received approximately a year of treatment at Motherlode University, Red Wing. He has not received treatment since that time. James reported that the severity of his stuttering fluctuates depending on his mood, and it is more pronounced in stressful situations.

He reported increased frequency of stuttering when he speaks to strangers, his instructors, and his father. He thought he was less dysfluent when he speaks to his mother, brother, sister, and close friends. He said that he would rather not order at restaurants, buy tickets at counters, introduce himself, or answer telephone calls. He did not think that he has difficulty with specific words or sounds.

Family and Social History

James is the oldest of three children. His younger brother and younger sister do not have communication problems. He believes that his maternal uncle and his son both stutter. James is not aware of any person on his father's side who stutters.

James lives with a roommate in a dorm on the campus. He says that his verbal interactions with his roommate are limited. He spends more time with his other friends. Reportedly, he has difficulty asking for dates because he is worried that he might stutter badly.

 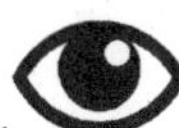

Educational and Occupational History

James has had part-time jobs in various businesses. He said that his stuttering was always a frustrating problem in the workplace. He usually avoided speaking to his supervisors. He tended to seek work that did not involve much oral communication.

James is studying for a degree in computer science. He is doing well in his courses. He does not think that his stuttering has negatively affected his coursework or relationship with his instructors. He plans to work for a private company when he finishes his degree. He is concerned about being able to communicate under job pressure. James appeared to be highly motivated for treatment, as he wants to be able to speak fluently.

Assessment Information

Orofacial Examination

An orofacial examination was performed to assess the structural and functional integrity of the oral mechanism. The examination did not reveal anything of clinical significance.

Types and Frequency of Dysfluencies

To analyze the types and the frequency of dysfluencies, a conversational speech sample was recorded. James was also asked to bring an audio-recorded conversational speech sample within the next 3 days. An analysis of the two samples revealed the following types and frequency of dysfluencies.

	Clinic Sample Total Words: 1,231	**Home Sample Total Words: 1,071**
Dysfluency Types	**Frequency of Dysfluency**	**Frequency of Dysfluency**
Interjections	86	26
Pauses	29	9
Part-word reps	68	60
Whole-word reps	9	57
Audible prolongations	52	4
Silent prolongations	7	4
Revisions	8	6
Incomplete phrases	2	1
Total	**261**	**167**
Percent Dysfluency Rate	**21**	**15.6**

Both of the speech samples contained pauses from 5 to 25 sec in duration. His sound and silent prolongations typically exceeded 1 sec. James's rate of speech was calculated between 110 and 150 words per minute depending on the amount and duration of pauses and prolongations. He intermittently rushed groups of words. Overall rate of speech was variable depending on number of dysfluencies.

An occasional eye blink and hand movements associated with dysfluencies were observed during the interview. These motor behaviors were most often associated with part-word repetitions and silent and sound prolongations.

Speech and Language Production and Language Comprehension

An informal assessment of a 100-utterance, 1,231-word, conversational speech and language sample did not reveal any speech sound production errors or expressive language problems. Therefore, these skills were judged appropriate for his level of education. No language comprehension problems were noted during the interview.

Voice

James spoke with laryngeal tension and hard glottal attack approximately 50% of the time. Tension and abrupt initiation of voice were often associated with dysfluencies. Nonetheless, he exhibited appropriate vocal intensity, intonation, and inflectional patterns.

Hearing Screening

Using the Grason Stadler ES3S Audiometer, James's hearing was screened bilaterally at 25 dB HL for 500, 1000, 2000, and 4000 Hz. He responded to all frequencies.

Diagnostic Summary

Analysis of the conversational speech samples revealed that James Foxx exhibited a severe fluency disorder with 18% to 21% dysfluency rates. His dominant dysfluencies were repetitions, prolongations, interjections, and pauses.

Recommendations

It is recommended that James Foxx receive treatment for his stuttering. With treatment, prognosis for fluent speech is judged to be good, as a brief duration of trial therapy suggested that stuttering may be eliminated with recommended fluency skills. The fluency-shaping program with the following treatment targets are recommended for James:

- appropriate airflow, rate reduction, and gentle phonatory onset
- production of 98% fluent speech within the clinic
- maintenance of at least 95% fluency in extraclinical situations

Submitted By ______________________________
Meena Wong, BA
Student Clinician

Client's Signature ______________________________
James Foxx

Approved By ______________________________
Nancy Lopez, MA, CCC-SLP
Speech-Language Pathologist
Clinical Supervisor

C.4. Practice in Diagnostic Report Writing

In practicing diagnostic report writing in the next section, use the information given on the left-hand pages, and write your report on the right-hand pages. Give appropriate headings and subheadings. Invent missing information.

Take note that the information on the left-hand pages is often written in an abbreviated style. Do not copy these truncated constructions. Instead, use the information to write formal, well-connected, sentences.

C.4.1. Practice Writing Diagnostic Report: *Speech Sound Disorder*

Data Sheet. Use these data to write your report on the opposite page. Use the correct headings.

Name of the clinic, city, and state: (invent)

> Write the name and address of the clinic.
>
> What kind of report?

Diagnostic Report

Mathew Moon, client; age, 8 years; address: (invent); telephone: (invent); clinician: yourself; date of assessment: (invent); diagnosis: articulation disorder; referred by: Dr. Lydia Bong, a counselor.

> **(L1H)**
>
> Identifying information
>
> Arrange appropriately

Background and Reasons for Referral

Use the previous information

No prior assessment at this facility

Informant: Mr. Sonny Moon, father

Date seen and evaluated (invent)

> **(L1H)**
>
> Who, how old a person, referred when, to which clinic, and why?

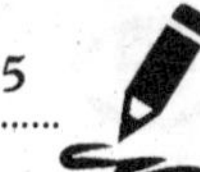

Write your report. Use the information on the data sheet. Invent information as needed.

Data Sheet. Use these data to write your report on the opposite page. Use the correct headings.

History

(L1H)

Birth and Development

(L2H)

Normal pregnancy, cesarean delivery

No other prenatal or natal complications

Normal infancy

Delayed motor development, but no specific information

First words at 18 months

Soon language development somewhat accelerated to approximate the normal.

Prenatal, birth

Mother's health

Early development

Early language development

Medical History

(L2H)

Major illnesses

Frequent middle ear infections; frequent medical treatment

Mild conductive hearing loss according to previous clinical reports

Frequent attacks of cold and allergies

Chicken pox at age 4 years

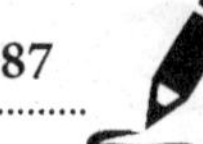

Write your report. Use the information on the data sheet. Invent information as needed.

Data Sheet. Use these data to write your report on the opposite page. Use the correct headings.

Family, Social, and Educational History

	(L2H)
An older brother (10 years), a younger sister (2 years)	Family How many children?
None with a communicative disorder	Any family history of communicative problems?
Mother: college graduate; a real estate broker Father: high school graduate; car repairman	Parents' education and occupation
Mathew, in second grade, doing below average schoolwork, was held back the first year in school	Educational information
He plays well with other children.	Child's companions and social behavior
Parents say he is cooperative, affectionate, and well behaved. Gets group speech treatment at his school once a week for 20 minutes.	Any other information about the family

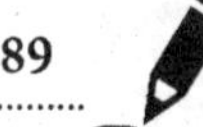

Write your report. Use the information on the data sheet. Invent information as needed.

Data Sheet. Use these data to write your report on the opposite page. Use the correct headings.

Assessment Information

Orofacial Examination

Class II malocclusion

Sluggish lingual movements

No other findings of significance

(L1H)

(L2H)

Describe the orofacial examination: integrity of oral and facial structures.

Give a general description of the face, mouth, teeth, tongue, hard and soft palate, and movement of the soft palate and the tongue.

Hearing Screening

Screened: 500, 1000, 2000, and 4000 Hz at 25 dB HL (Maico MA25)

Failed at all tested frequencies.

Needs a complete audiological examination; will be referred to an audiologist

(L2H)

What frequencies were screened and at what level?

What were the results?

Write your report. Use the information on the data sheet. Invent information as needed.

Data Sheet. Use these data to write your report on the opposite page. Use the correct headings.

Speech Sound Production and Intelligibility

Conversational speech sample

Goldman–Fristoe Test of Articulation

Numerous errors in both

In the initial position of words, omitted: /b, d, p, f, v, r, k/; substituted: t/k; distorted: /z, s/

In the medial position of words, omitted: /b, m, f, z, s, l, g, r/

In the final position of words, omitted: /b, d, p, f, v, r, k, t, l, m, n, s/

The same errors in conversational speech

Intelligibility with contextual cues: 60% for utterances

(L2H)

How was speech sound production assessed?

Give the full name of tests administered. Do not ignore speech samples.

Summarize the errors in a table.

What was the speech intelligibility?

Write your report. Use the information on the data sheet. Invent information as needed.

Data Sheet. Use these data to write your report on the opposite page. Use the correct headings.

Language Production and Comprehension

Speech-language sample: 120 utterances

MLU: 3.0 words

Analysis of conversational speech for missing grammatical features

Many morphological features missing, but consider the errors of articulation

(invent missing morphological features, including the regular plural, possessive, prepositions)

Limited sentence structures

Tests administered:

Peabody Picture Vocabulary Test (3rd ed.; PPVT III), Form A

Results: Raw score, 108; standard score, 100; percentile, 50; age equivalency, 8–0.

Expressive Vocabulary Test (EVT)

Results: Raw score, 80; standard score, 101; percentile, 53; age equivalency, 8–2.

(L2H)

How did you assess language production?

How did you analyze the results?

What were the results of the analysis?

How did you assess comprehension?

What were the results?

Voice and Fluency

Informally assessed through conversational speech samples

Judged to be within normal limits

(L2H)

How did you assess voice and fluency?

What is your evaluation?

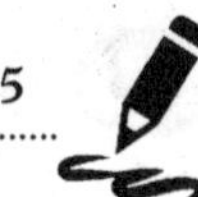

Write your report. Use the information on the data sheet. Invent information as needed.

Data Sheet. Use these data to write your report on the opposite page. Use the correct headings.

Diagnostic Summary

Multiple misarticulations

Speech intelligibility: 60%

Normal voice and fluency

Limited language structures; many missing morphological features

(L1H)

Summarize the communicative problems.

Recommendations

Treatment recommended

With treatment, good prognosis

Goal is to teach the misarticulated phonemes. A more detailed language assessment later.

A program to train parents in maintenance techniques

An audiological assessment

Submitted By ______________________

Parent's Signature ______________________

Approved By ______________________

(L1H)

Do you recommend treatment?

What are the priority treatment targets?

Who submitted the report?

Write the name, degree, and title.

Parent's name and signature.

Who approved the report?

Write the name, degree, certification, and title of a clinical supervisor.

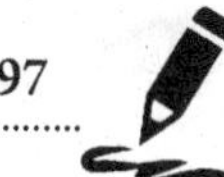

Write your report. Use the information on the data sheet. Invent information as needed.

C.4.2. Practice Writing Diagnostic Report: *Child Language Disorder*

Data Sheet. Use these data to write your report on the opposite page. Use the correct headings.

Name of the clinic, city, and state: (invent)

Write the name and address of the clinic.

Diagnostic Report

Sylvia Sun, client; age, 5 years, 2 months; address: (invent); telephone: (invent); clinician: yourself; date of assessment: (invent); diagnosis: Language Disorder; referred by: Dr. Chang Loongson, a physician

(L1H)

What kind of report?

Identifying information

Arrange appropriately

Background and Reasons for Referral

Date seen at the clinic (invent)

Use the previous information

No prior assessment at this facility

Informant: Mrs. Katie Sun, mother

(L1H)

Who, how old a person, referred when, to which clinic, and why?

Write your report. Use the information on the data sheet. Invent information as needed.

Data Sheet. Use these data to write your report on the opposite page. Use the correct headings.

History

Birth and Development

Normal pregnancy, delivery

No significant prenatal or natal complications

Normal infancy

Delayed language and motor development

First words at 22 months

Two-word phrases not until 28 months

Errors of articulation

"Does not speak in complete sentences" (mother)

"Does not know many words" (mother)

(L1H)

(L2H)

Prenatal, birth

Mother's health

Early development

Early language development

Medical History

One episode of high fever and convulsions at age 16 months

Prone to frequent episodes of coughs, colds, and allergic reactions

Chicken pox at age 4 years

Slow physical growth

(L2H)

Diseases of significance

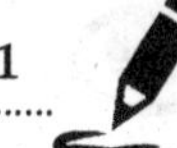

Write your report. Use the information on the data sheet. Invent information as needed.

Data Sheet. Use these data to write your report on the opposite page. Use the correct headings.

Family, Social, and Educational History

	(L2H)
An older sister (8 years), a younger brother (3 years)	Family
Sister diagnosed with intellectual disabilities, enrolled in special education	How many children?
No parental concern about the younger brother's speech and language	
Older sister: language delayed, getting treated in school	Any family history of communicative problems?
Mother: a high school graduate; a receptionist in an auto body repair shop Father: high school graduate; plumber	Parent's education and occupation
Enrolled in a kindergarten program Needs special attention	Educational information
Does not play cooperatively Has a few companions who are much younger	Child's companions and social behavior
	Any other information about the family

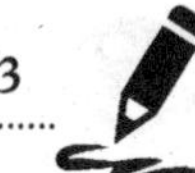

Write your report. Use the information on the data sheet. Invent information as needed.

Data Sheet. Use these data to write your report on the opposite page. Use the correct headings.

Assessment Information

Orofacial Examination

No malocclusion

Sluggish lingual movements

Slow diadochokinetic rate

No other findings of significance

(L1H)

(L2H)

Describe the orofacial examination: integrity of oral and facial structures.

Give a general description of the face, mouth, teeth, tongue, hard and soft palate, and movement of the soft palate and the tongue.

Hearing Screening

Screened: 500, 1000, 2000, and 4000 Hz at 25 dB HL (Maico Pilot Test Audiometer)

Passed at all tested frequencies

(L2H)

What frequencies were screened and at what level?

What were the results?

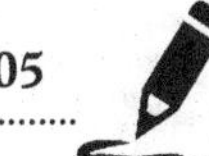

Write your report. Use the information on the data sheet. Invent information as needed.

Data Sheet. Use these data to write your report on the opposite page. Use the correct headings.

Speech Sound Production and Speech Intelligibility

Conversational speech sample

Goldman–Fristoe Test of Articulation: Second Edition

Numerous errors in both

In the initial position of words, omitted: /b, d, t, l, g, m, n, k/; distorted: /z, s/

In the medial position of words, omitted: /b, m, f, z, s, l, g, r/

In the final position of words, omitted: /b, d, p, r, k, t, m, n, s/

The same errors in conversational speech

Intelligibility with contextual cues: 80% for utterances

(L2H)

How was speech production assessed?

Give the full name of tests administered. Do not ignore speech samples.

Summarize the errors in a table.

What was the speech intelligibility?

Write your report. Use the information on the data sheet. Invent information as needed.

Data Sheet. Use these data to write your report on the opposite page. Use the correct headings.

Language Production and Comprehension

Language sample: 60 utterances

Shown pictures, objects, and toys to evoke language

MLU: 4.0 words

Analysis of conversational speech for missing grammatical features and pragmatic functions

Limited vocabulary

Many morphological features missing (invent missing morphological features, e.g., the plural *s*, present progressive *ing*, past tense *ed*)

Typically, three- to four-word utterances

Few grammatically complete sentences

Limited sentence structures and few sentence varieties

Difficulty in maintaining topic and in conversational turn taking

Tests administered:

Receptive One-Word Picture Vocabulary Test (ROWPVT)

Results: Raw score, 46; standard score, 85; percentile, 16; age equivalency, 4–0

Expressive One-Word Picture Vocabulary Test (EOWPVT)

Results: Raw score, 40; standard score, 82; percentile, 11; age equivalency, 3–10

Clinical judgment during interview and language sampling

Comprehension of conversational speech: Approximately that of a 3-year-old

(L2H)

How did you assess language production?

What tests?

How did you analyze the results?

What were the results of the analysis?

How did you assess language comprehension?

What were the results?

Voice and Fluency

Informally assessed through conversational speech samples

Limited fluency because of limited language

Voice judged to be within normal limits

(L2H)

How did you assess voice and fluency?

What is your evaluation?

Write your report. Use the information on the data sheet. Invent information as needed.

Data Sheet. Use these data to write your report on the opposite page. Use the correct headings.

Diagnostic Summary

Multiple sound errors

Speech intelligibility: 80%

Normal voice but limited fluency

Limited vocabulary and language structures; many missing morphological features; pragmatic problems; deficiency in language comprehension

(L1H)

Summarize the communicative problems.

Recommendations

Treatment recommended

With treatment, good prognosis

Initial goal is to expand vocabulary, teach early morphemes and basic sentence structures.

Later goal is to teach correct articulation of phonemes, pragmatic features.

A more detailed language assessment before initiating treatment

Parent training in a home treatment and maintenance program

(L1H)

Do you recommend treatment?

What are the priority treatment targets?

Submitted By ______________________________

Who submitted the report?

Write the name, degree, and title.

Parent's Signature ______________________________
Mrs. Katie Sun

Parent's name and signature

Approved By ______________________________

Who approved the report?

Write the name, degree, certification, and titles of a clinical supervisor.

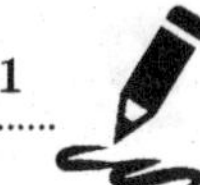

Write your report. Use the information on the data sheet. Invent information as needed.

C.4.3. Practice Writing Diagnostic Report: *Stuttering*

Data Sheet. Use these data to write your report on the opposite page. Use the correct headings.

Name of the clinic, city, and state: (invent)

Write the name and address of the clinic.

Diagnostic Report

Marvin Lenson, client; age, 32 years; address: (invent); telephone: (invent); clinician: yourself; date of assessment: (invent); diagnosis: stuttering; referral: self

(L1H)

What kind of report?

Identifying information

Arrange appropriately

Background and Reasons for Referral

Use the previous information

Date evaluated (invent)

Several prior assessments and treatments at various clinics with no lasting effects

Informant: Self

Client reported that: stuttering started when he was about 5 years old (according to his mother)

Has had prior treatment throughout the school years

Does not recall treatment techniques except that he was encouraged to think before talking

Frequency of stuttering varies across situations; but more when talking to strangers and his boss; more fluent talking to wife; avoids telephones, ordering in restaurants, and talking to groups

(L1H)

Who, how old a person, referred when, to which clinic, and why?

Summarize the history of stuttering.

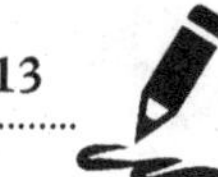

Write your report. Use the information on the data sheet. Invent information as needed.

Data Sheet. Use these data to write your report on the opposite page. Use the correct headings.

History

(L1H)

Birth and Development

(L2H)

Prenatal, birth

Mother had told the client that everything was normal.

Mother's health

Mother's health during pregnancy reportedly normal

Early development

Normal infancy

Normal motor development

Early language development

Advanced early language development, as told by parents

Considers himself verbally competent; likes to read and write; has good vocabulary and command of the language.

Medical History

(L2H)

Diseases of significance

Nothing of clinical significance

Note: In the case of most adult clients, *Birth and Development* may not be a necessary heading. However, when information that is relevant for a given disorder is available, it should be included.

Write your report. Use the information on the data sheet. Invent information as needed.

Data Sheet. Use these data to write your report on the opposite page. Use the correct headings.

Family, Social, and Educational History

(L2H)

An older brother (37 years), a younger sister (27 years), a younger brother (24 years)

Older brother used to stutter but has been mostly fluent for the past 10 years; has had unspecified treatment.

A maternal uncle (65 years old) still stutters.

A paternal aunt (62 years old) used to stutter but has been fluent for many years. Has no family history of other communication disorders

Family

How many children?

Any family history of communicative problems?

Both parents hold doctoral degrees; Mother: a pediatrician; Father: a clinical psychologist

Parents' education and occupation

Client holds a master's degree in structural engineering. Works for a construction company

Educational and occupational information

Married; wife owns a clothing store

One daughter (3 years old), no concerns with her speech or language

Personal information

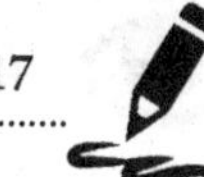

Write your report. Use the information on the data sheet. Invent information as needed.

Data Sheet. Use these data to write your report on the opposite page. Use the correct headings.

Assessment Information

> (L1H)
>
> (L2H)
>
> Describe the orofacial examination: integrity of oral and facial structures.

Orofacial Examination

Nothing of clinical significance

> (L2H)
>
> What frequencies were screened and at what level?
>
> What were the results?

Hearing Screening

Screened: 500, 1000, 2000, and 4000 Hz at 25 dB HL (Earscan 3 ES3S Audiometer)

Passed the screening

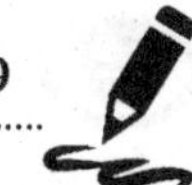

Write your report. Use the information on the data sheet. Invent information as needed.

Data Sheet. Use these data to write your report on the opposite page. Use the correct headings.

Speech and Language Production

Informally assessed as the client was interviewed

Judged to have normal articulation and superior language skills

Speech intelligibility was 100% for utterances with or without knowledge of contexts.

(L2H)

How were speech and language production assessed?

What was the speech intelligibility?

Summarize the observations.

Voice

Informally assessed as the client was interviewed

Vocal qualities judged to be normal

(L2H)

How assessed?

Summarize the observations.

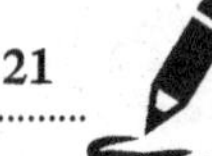

Write your report. Use the information on the data sheet. Invent information as needed.

Data Sheet. Use these data to write your report on the opposite page. Use the correct headings.

Assessment of Fluency

Conversational speech sample: 2,000 words

Oral reading sample: 500 words

Two home samples of at least 1,000 words each requested for later analysis

Analysis of types and frequency of dysfluencies (all types)

Calculation of percent dysfluency based on the number of words spoken

Results:

In conversational speech:

Part-word reps, 57; sound prolongations, 48; syllable interjections, 28; whole-word reps, 39; pauses (1 s or more), 45; broken words, 21

Total number of dysfluencies: 238

Percent dysfluency: 11.9

Oral reading:

Part-word reps: 42; sound prolongations: 39; syllable interjections: 34; whole-word reps: 53; pauses (1 s or more): 54; broken words: 21

Total number of dysfluencies: 243

Percent dysfluency: 48.6

Eye blinks, knitting of the eyebrows associated with sound prolongations and word repetitions

(L2H)

How did you assess fluency and stuttering?

How did you analyze the results?

What were the results of the analysis?

Describe the frequency and types of dysfluencies in oral reading

Describe the associated motor behaviors

Write your report. Use the information on the data sheet. Invent information as needed.

Data Sheet. Use these data to write your report on the opposite page. Use the correct headings.

Diagnostic Summary

Clinically significant percentage of dysfluency: 11.9%

Part-word reps, sound prolongations, syllable interjections, whole-word reps, pauses, and broken words

Higher frequency of dysfluency in oral reading: 48.6

Few associated motor behaviors

(L1H)

Summarize the dysfluency rates.

Specify the types.

Recommendations

Treatment recommended

With treatment, judged prognosis is favorable

Goal is to teach the skills of fluency (gentle phonatory onset, rate reduction through syllable prolongation, and appropriate airflow management)

Self-monitoring skills for maintenance

Submitted By ______________________________

Client's Signature ___________________________
Marvin Lenson

Approved By ______________________________

(L1H)

Do you recommend treatment?

What are the priority treatment targets?

Who submitted the report?

Write the name, degree, and title.

Client's name and signature

Who approved the report?

Write the name, degree, certification, and titles of a clinical supervisor.

Write your report. Use the information on the data sheet. Invent information as needed.

C.4.4. Practice Writing Diagnostic Report: *Voice Disorder*

Data Sheet. Use these data to write your report on the opposite page. Use the correct headings.

Name of the clinic, city, and state (invent)

Write the name and address of the clinic.

Diagnostic Report

Raj Mohan, 35 years old; address: (invent); telephone: (invent); clinician: yourself; date of assessment: (invent); diagnosis: Voice Disorder (Inadequate Loudness); referred by: Dr. Melanie Mallard, an otolaryngologist.

(L1H)

What kind of report?

Identifying information

Arrange appropriately

Background and Reasons for Referral

Use the previous information

No prior assessment; date assessed (invent)

Informant: Self

Client reports that: his voice is too soft for his occupation (high school teacher); voice gets tired too soon during the working days; students complain because of too soft voice; has had the problem for the past 2 years; not much variation
[Insert Page Break]

(L1H)

Who, how old a person, referred when, to which clinic, and why?

Summarize the history of the voice disorder.

Write your report. Use the information on the data sheet. Invent information as needed.

Data Sheet. Use these data to write your report on the opposite page. Use the correct headings.

History

(L1H)

Birth and Development

(L2H)

No relevant information; eliminate this heading in the report

Medical History

(L2H)

Ear, Nose, and Throat (ENT) specialist's report negative; normal laryngeal structures

Diseases of significance

No medical basis for the symptoms

ENT recommends voice treatment.

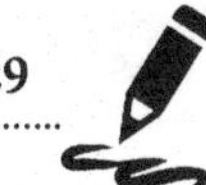

Write your report. Use the information on the data sheet. Invent information as needed.

Data Sheet. Use these data to write your report on the opposite page. Use the correct headings.

Family, Social, and Educational History

The only child in the family

No history of voice disorder or other communication problems

Mother: college graduate; a college counselor

Father: college graduate; a college admissions officer

(L2H)

Family
How many children?

Any family history of communicative problems?

Parents' education and occupation

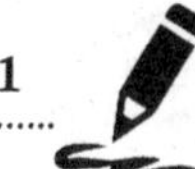

Write your report. Use the information on the data sheet. Invent information as needed.

Data Sheet. Use these data to write your report on the opposite page. Use the correct headings.

Assessment Information

(L1H)

(L2H)

Describe the orofacial examination: integrity of oral and facial structures.

Orofacial Examination

Negative (nothing of clinical significance)

(L2H)

What frequencies were screened and at what level?

What were the results?

Hearing Screening

Screened: 500, 1000, 2000, and 4000 Hz at 25 dB HL (Grason Stadler GS18 Audiometer)

Passed at all frequencies

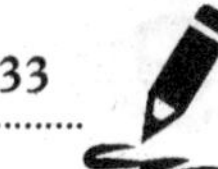

Write your report. Use the information on the data sheet. Invent information as needed.

Data Sheet. Use these data to write your report on the opposite page. Use the correct headings.

Speech, Language, and Fluency

Based on the observation of conversational speech during interview, judged to be within normal limits

Speech 100% intelligible with or without contextual knowledge

(L2H)

How were they assessed?

What was the speech intelligibility?

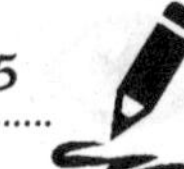

Write your report. Use the information on the data sheet. Invent information as needed.

Data Sheet. Use these data to write your report on the opposite page. Use the correct headings.

Voice

Subjectively rated on a 5-point scale from very soft to very loud (1 = very soft; 5 = very loud)

Received a rating of 2, soft voice

Also measured with a sound level meter with the microphone placed at 8 in. from the client's face

Measurement showed 45 dB, judged too soft

Additional data: in each class period, the client's students request some five to six times to speak louder

Was asked to baserate the frequency with which the students request him to speak louder over 5 consecutive days

(L2H)

How was voice assessed?

What were the results?

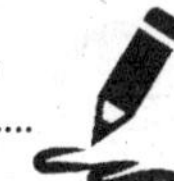

Write your report. Use the information on the data sheet. Invent information as needed.

Data Sheet. Use these data to write your report on the opposite page. Use the correct headings.

Diagnostic Summary

Self-report, clinical judgment, and instrumental measurement suggest a voice that is too soft to meet the demands of the client's social and occupational life.

(L1H)

Summarize the voice disorder.

Recommendations

Treatment recommended

With treatment, good prognosis

Shape a louder voice considered appropriate for classroom teaching

Reduce or eliminate the number of student requests to speak louder by shaping appropriately louder voice

(L1H)

Do you recommend treatment?

What are the priority treatment targets?

Submitted By ________________________________

Who submitted the report?

Write the name, degree, and title.

Client's Signature ______________________________

Raj Mohan

Client's name and signature

Approved By ________________________________

Who approved the report?

Write the name, degree, certification, and titles of a clinical supervisor.

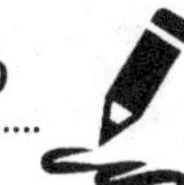

Write your report. Use the information on the data sheet. Invent information as needed.

Note to Student Clinicians

Contact your clinic secretary for additional examples of assessment reports. Take note of variations in formats. Practice writing reports according to your clinic format. Use the practice formats presented in this section.

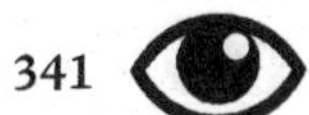

C.5. Comprehensive Treatment Plans

Treatment plans written for clients vary across professional settings. The plans written in university clinics are perhaps more detailed than those that are written in other settings. A student who learns to write detailed and comprehensive treatment plans can easily write briefer reports; but a student who has written only brief reports in incomplete sentences will find it hard to write longer, comprehensive reports. Therefore, this section gives examples of more and less detailed treatment plans.

Treatment plans, like assessment reports, need not follow the format of the *Publication Manual of the American Psychological Association* (APA *Manual*, APA style) in every respect. Heading styles will vary; the examples that follow use different styles to illustrate this variety. One-sentence paragraphs, lists (incomplete sentences), and other deviations from the APA style may be acceptable in treatment plans, especially in those that are brief.

Student clinicians are encouraged to see these varied forms and styles to learn about practice across clinics. The variations should not be thought of as inconsistencies. Student clinicians need to find out the accepted format in their clinic by talking to their clinic director and clinical supervisor.

On the following page, we begin with an exemplar of a comprehensive treatment plan that is more detailed than brief treatment plans and may include the following:

- a brief summary of previous assessment data
- treatment targets
- treatment and probe procedures
- maintenance program
- follow-up and booster treatment procedures

A student who writes a comprehensive treatment plan understands the total management program for a client. The student may or may not complete the program in a semester or quarter. Nonetheless, writing a comprehensive treatment program is a good exercise in visualizing the entire treatment sequence from the beginning to the end, which goes beyond clinical practicum to what clinicians do in professional settings. After assessing their clients, clinicians develop comprehensive treatment plans for them. Therefore, although the student clinicians implement only a portion of a treatment plan, it is desirable to think of the total program for a client.

C.5.1. Comprehensive Treatment Plan: *Speech Sound Disorder*

University Speech and Hearing Clinic

Treatment Plan

Name: Oliver Driver | Diagnosis: Articulation Disorder

Date of Birth: xx-xx-xxxx | File No.: 900111-3

Address: | Semesters in Therapy: 1

City: | Date of Report: xx-xx-xxxx

School: University Preschool | Telephone: 222-782-9832

Background Information

Oliver Driver, a 4-year-old male child, began his first semester of speech treatment at the University Speech and Hearing Clinic on [xx/xx/xxxx]. Oliver's speech and language were evaluated on [xx/xx/xxxx]. The evaluation revealed a speech sound disorder characterized by substitutions, omissions, and reduced intelligibility. See his folder for a diagnostic report.

Treatment was recommended to teach correct productions of misarticulated phonemes to increase speech intelligibility. Based on Oliver's cooperative behavior during assessment, prognosis for improved articulation was judged as good.

Target Behaviors

The **final target** for Oliver is to produce all phonemes correctly in conversational speech with at least 90% accuracy.

The **initial target** is to produce selected phonemes correctly. Based on their inconsistent production during assessment, the following phonemes were selected for the initial treatment: /p/, /m/, /s/, /k/, and /g/. Production of each phoneme was baserated with 20 stimulus words administered on modeled and evoked discrete trials with the following correct baseline response rates:

Phonemes	Evoked (%)	Modeled (%)
/p/	15	17
/m/	10	24
/s/	12	22
/k/	18	20
/g/	14	17

Treatment began after the baserates were obtained. The following general treatment procedures will be used during the semester. The procedures will be modified as suggested by Oliver's performance data. These changes will be described in the final progress report.

Treatment and Probe Procedures

Each target phoneme will initially be trained at the word level. When Oliver's probe response rate at the word level meets a 90% correct criterion, training will be initiated on two-word phrases. A similar probe criterion will be used to shift training to sentences and then to conversational speech.

Intermixed probes in which trained and untrained words, phrases, or sentences are alternated will be administered every time Oliver meets a tentative training criterion of 90% correct response rate on a block of 20 evoked training trials. Oliver will be trained to meet this criterion at each level of response topography (words, phrases, and sentences).

Initially, the clinician will provide stimulus pictures. Subsequently, Oliver will be required to find at least five pictures in magazines that represent the target sound and bring them to the clinic sessions. After he correctly produces a target sound on five consecutive trials, he will paste a picture that represents the just-trained sound in a book. This book will be used for both clinic and home practice.

Intervention will begin at each level with discrete trials and modeling. The clinician will show Oliver a picture, ask a question ("What is this?"), and model the response (word or phrase). Oliver will then be required to imitate the clinician's production. When Oliver correctly imitates the target sound on five consecutive trials, modeling will be discontinued. The clinician will show Oliver a picture and ask, "What is this?" to evoke a response.

At the modeled and evoked word levels, verbal reinforcement will be administered on an FR1 schedule for correct productions. At the phrase and sentence levels, an FR4 schedule will be used. At the conversational level, verbal reinforcement will be delivered on an approximate VR5 schedule. All incorrect productions at each level will immediately be interrupted by saying, "stop."

Modeling will be reintroduced if Oliver gives two to four incorrect responses on the evoked trials. Shaping with manual guidance will be used as necessary.

The clinician will chart all productions in all treatment sessions. Oliver also will chart productions with an X under the *happy face* (correct responses) or X under the *sad face* (incorrect responses). At the end of each session, Oliver will assist the clinician in recording his progress on a graph.

It is expected that different target sounds will reach the training criterion at different times. Therefore, the clinician expects to train several sounds at different response topographies in each session. Some sounds may be trained at the word level, whereas others may be trained at the phrase or even sentence level. When the initially selected target sounds meet the criterion of a 90% correct probe rate in conversational speech in the clinic, new target sounds will be baserated and trained.

Maintenance Program

After Oliver produces the target sound with 90% accuracy at the evoked word level, his mother, Mrs. Janice Driver, will be asked to participate in treatment. Initially, she will observe the treatment procedure. Soon, Mrs. Driver will be taught to present stimulus items and chart correct and incorrect productions. She will be taught to immediately reinforce the correct productions and stop Oliver at the earliest sign of an inaccurate production.

After Oliver's mother identifies correct and incorrect responses with at least 80% accuracy in the clinic session, she will be taught to work with him at home. Mrs. Driver will begin with such structured activities as reciting from a list or reading from the book that Oliver will be developing in treatment. Assignments will progress to monitoring and recording speech during dinner and phone conversations with Oliver's grandmother, who will be encouraged to prompt and then praise the correct productions. The clinician, Oliver, and his mother will review tape-recorded home assignments. The mother will be given feedback on the procedures implemented at home.

When Oliver produces the target sound with 90% accuracy in conversation in the sessions, he will be taken out of the clinic to practice correct productions in nonclinical situations. The clinician will take Oliver for a walk on campus and talk with him. Subsequently, he may be taken to the campus bookstore, library, cafeteria, and other places. Eventually, his speech may be monitored informally in shopping centers and restaurants.

When Oliver's speech is 98% intelligible and his sound productions are 90% correct, he may be dismissed from treatment. A follow-up visit will be scheduled for 6 months after dismissal. Based on the initial follow-up results, booster treatment, treatment for persistent errors, or additional follow-up assessments will be planned.

Submitted By ____
Marla Model, BA
Student Clinician

Client's Signature ____
Mrs. Janice Driver

Approved By ____
Barbara Sierra, MS, CCC/SLP
Speech-Language Pathologist
Clinical Supervisor

C.6. Brief Treatment Plans

Brief or short-term treatment plans, also known as lesson plans, are probably used more frequently than longer ones. The scope of these plans varies across clinics and supervisors. Some plans describe what will be done in only a session or two. Others might describe treatment objectives and procedures planned for a week, a quarter, or a semester. Even those that describe the plan for a semester may not be as comprehensive as a complete treatment plan. In some plans, only the treatment objectives may be listed.

However, all treatment plans—long or short—should contain a statement of prognosis and a description of target behaviors, treatment procedures, and performance criteria.

The examples of brief treatment plans given on the following pages show slightly different formats in which they can be written. The sampling of formats is not comprehensive; the examples suggest a few basic variations. Heading styles and paragraph formats are varied purposefully.

C.6.1. Brief Treatment Plan: *Stuttering*

Speech and Hearing Clinic
Eastern State University
Bedford, California

Jazmin Jimenez, a 6-year-old girl, was seen on February x, xxxx, for a speech assessment at the Speech and Hearing Clinic of Eastern State University, Bedford, California. Assessment results showed that Jazmin stuttered with a dysfluency rate of 11% in conversational speech. Her dysfluencies were characterized by repetitions, prolongations, pauses, interjections, and revisions. Treatment was recommended. With consistent treatment, prognosis for improved fluency was judged to be good.

A response cost procedure was used. Jazmin's fluent speech intervals were reinforced with a token backed up by a tangible reinforcer. Each dysfluency resulted in a loss of token, and the accumulated tokens were exchanged for a small gift she had selected at the beginning of each session.

Final Treatment Objective: A dysfluency rate that does not exceed 5% in Jazmin's home and in other nonclinical settings

Target Behaviors

- **Increased frequency of fluent utterances in conversational speech.** In the beginning sessions, the fluent utterances will be words or phrases spoken at Jazmin's typical rate. Subsequently, longer phrases and sentences will be the target behaviors.
- **Decreased frequency of dysfluencies**. Reduction of dysfluencies to 2% of the spoken words or less.

Treatment Procedures

The clinician will

- Establish a baseline of dysfluency and speech rates in conversational speech before starting treatment.
- Begin treatment at the level of words and short phrases.
- Reinforce Jazmin's fluent utterances with both verbal praise and a token on a fixed ratio of 1 (FR1, every target response reinforced).
- Increase the length of target utterances as Jazmin sustains 98% stutter-free speech at each level of response complexity.
- Instruct and model target responses consistently in the beginning stages and as often as necessary in subsequent stages of treatment; eventually fade the instructions and modeling.
- Give corrective feedback for each dysfluency and while doing this, withdraw a token Jazmin had earned.
- Initiate fluency maintenance procedures when Jazmin sustains no more than a 2% dysfluency in conversational speech across three sessions. Jazmin's parents will receive training in verbally reinforcing their daughter's fluent utterances.
- Take Jazmin to extraclinical situations to evoke and verbally reinforce fluent speech.
- Analyze home speech samples to judge maintenance of fluency.
- Schedule follow-up for 3, 6, and 12 months postdismissal.
- Arrange booster treatment as needed.

Signed ______________________________

Gloria Marquez, BA
Student Clinician

I understand the results of the evaluation and agree to the recommended treatment plan.

Signed ______________________________ Date ____________________

Sofia Jimenez, Mother

____

Henriette Borden, PhD, CCC-SLP
Speech-Language Pathologist
Clinical Supervisor

C.6.2. Brief Treatment Plan: *Speech Sound Disorder*

Valley Speech and Hearing Center
Nordstrom, Maine

Rudy Amos, a 7-year and 3-month-old boy, was referred to the Valley Speech and Hearing Center for assessment and treatment of a speech sound disorder. According to an assessment made on xx-xx-xxxx, Rudy's speech sound disorder is limited to omissions of the following phonemes in both the word initial and final positions: /k, l, s, t, r/ and /z/. Treatment was recommended. Prognosis for improvement was judged excellent because Rudy was readily stimulable and highly cooperative during a brief period of trial therapy.

The treatment began on xx-xx-xxxx. A baserate showed 0% to 10% accuracy on the target phonemes. The baserates on modeled and evoked trials were similar.

The treatment will have the following final goal, specific objectives, and procedures.

Final treatment goal: Correct production of target phonemes maintained in conversational speech produced in the natural environment with at least 90% accuracy.

Objective 1. Correct production of misarticulated phonemes in the initial, medial, and final word positions with a minimum of 90% accuracy.

Procedures: Pictures that help evoke words with the target sounds in all word positions will be used. Instructions, demonstrations, and visual feedback will be used, as found necessary. Modeling will be provided, and, if necessary, various sound-shaping techniques will be used to refine the imitated responses. Rudy will be verbally reinforced for progressively better imitations of modeled responses. Corrective feedback will be given for incorrect responses.

When Rudy meets the training criterion of 90% correct production of words for a block of 20 treatment trials, an intermixed probe will be conducted. Training and probe trials will be alternated until this criterion is met.

Objective 2. Correct production of misarticulated phonemes in phrases and sentences.

Procedures: Training will be shifted to phrase level when Rudy meets the probe criterion for words and to sentence level when his responses at the phrase level meet the probe criterion. Picture description and controlled conversation will be used to evoke target phrases and sentences. Modeling will be provided as needed. Correct responses will be reinforced on a variable schedule designed to progressively reduce the amount of feedback. Corrective feedback will be given for all incorrect responses.

Objective 3. Correct production of misarticulated phonemes in conversational speech with varied audiences.

Procedures: Initially, the clinician will evoke conversational speech and model and reinforce correct productions. When Rudy's accuracy of production in conversational speech reaches at least 80%, other persons will serve as the audience.

Objective 4. Correct production of target phonemes in extraclinical situations.

Procedures: Rudy will be taken out of the treatment room to various settings on the campus to strengthen the correct production of the target phonemes. Correct productions will be prompted and reinforced in a subtle manner in such places as the campus bookstore and restaurants.

Objective 5. Teaching Rudy's mother to evoke and reinforce correct productions in conversational speech at home.

Procedures: The mother will be asked to initially observe the sessions and later participate in the treatment sessions. Mrs. Amos will be taught to recognize the correct productions and to immediately praise Rudy. Mrs. Amos will be asked to hold brief and informal treatment sessions at home. Recorded home speech samples will be used to assess the correct production of phonemes at home.

The dismissal criterion: A 90% or better correct production of the target phonemes in conversational speech produced in extraclinical situations. Periodic home speech samples, recorded by the mother, will be used to assess this criterion.

The procedure will be modified as found necessary during the treatment sessions.

Follow-up evaluations will be conducted 3, 6, and 12 months after the dismissal. Booster treatment will be scheduled as needed.

Signed ________________________________

Mohamed Ali, MA, CCC-SLP
Speech-Language Pathologist

I understand the treatment program, and I agree to it.

Signed ________________________________

Ms. Lydia Amos
Mother

C.6.3. Brief Treatment Plan: *Child Language Disorder*

Speech and Hearing Clinic
Southern State University
Johnsonville, Louisiana

Timothy Krebs, a 4-year, 2-month-old boy, was evaluated at the Speech and Hearing Clinic at the Southern State University on x-x-xxxx. The evaluation revealed a severe language disorder. Case history and assessment data showed that his language performance is limited to a few words and phrases. A detailed assessment report can be found in Timothy's file. A language treatment program was recommended.

Timothy will be seen two times weekly in sessions lasting 45 min. His father, Mr. John Krebs, will accompany him to the clinic and will participate in treatment sessions. It is judged that prognosis for improved language performance is good if treatment is consistent and a home treatment and maintenance program is sustained. The following treatment objectives were selected for this semester [specify].

Initial Treatment Objective

Correct production of selected functional words at 90% accuracy.

With the help of Timothy's father, the following 20 targets consisting of single words or two-word phrases of high functional value were selected for initial treatment:

cup	sock	milk	shoe	Jenny (sister)
juice	more	eat	give me	walking
no more	I want	cookie	apple	bath
shirt	look!	Hi	Binny (dog)	John (friend)

Timothy did not produce any of these words on evoked or modeled baseline trials.

Subsequent Treatment Objectives

- correct production of additional words
- expansion of single words into phrases and sentences
- production of early morphological features (present progressive, regular plural, possessive, prepositions, pronouns, etc.)

Initial Treatment Procedures

- Pictures, objects, toys, acted-out situations, and role-playing will be used as stimuli to evoke the target words or phrases.
- The clinician and the father will take turns in evoking the target words or phrases.
- Initially, gross approximations will be reinforced by verbal praise and such natural reinforcers as handing an object, complying with a request, and so forth. Subsequently, only better approximations will be reinforced.
- All correct and incorrect productions will be measured in each treatment session.

- When single words meet the training criterion of 90% accuracy across two sessions, intermixed probes will be conducted to assess generalized production.
- Words that meet the 90% accurate probe criterion will be expanded into phrases, and phrases that meet the same probe criterion will be expanded into simple sentences.
- The father will be asked to conduct similar treatment sessions at home and bring recorded samples of sessions for evaluation and feedback.

Subsequent Treatment Procedures

- Additional words, selected in consultation with the father, will be trained using the same procedure described under initial treatment procedures.
- Additional words will be expanded into phrases and sentences.
- Selected morphological features will be initially trained in words and later expanded into phrases and sentences.

It is expected that Timothy will need extended treatment and that both the treatment objectives and procedures will be modified in light of his performance data. The father's participation in training from the beginning will help maintenance. A more complete maintenance program will be developed later.

Signed ______________________________
Trisha Muniz, BA
Student Clinician

I understand the results of the evaluation and agree to the recommended treatment plan.

Signed ______________________________
Mr. John Krebs

Signed ______________________________ Date ____________________
Maya Real, MA, CCC-SLP
Speech-Language Pathologist
Clinical Supervisor

C.6.4. Brief Treatment Plan: *Voice Disorder*

The Sunshine Speech and Hearing Center
Zingsville, Vermont

Roshana Hersh, a 21-year-old female college student, was seen at the Sunshine Speech and Hearing Center on xx-xx-xxxx, for a voice evaluation. The evaluation suggested a pattern of vocal abuse associated with a persistent hoarseness of voice, low pitch, and socially inappropriate intensity. Her vocal abuse consists mainly of excessive talking over the telephone and shouting at children she supervises as a teacher's aide in a kindergarten school. The detailed case history and assessment data can be found in her file. A treatment program to improve her voice quality was recommended. Considering her high degree of motivation for improvement that she expressed during the interview, prognosis with treatment for improved vocal quality was judged to be good.

Treatment Targets

Goal 1. Production of clear voice at least 90% of the time Roshana speaks by reducing the hoarseness of voice

Objective 1a. Reduced amount of talking over the phone

Objective 1b. Reduced amount of shouting at the school

Goal 2. Increased vocal pitch

Objective 2a. Higher pitch at the level of words and phrases

Objective 2b. Higher pitch at the level of conversational speech

Goal 3. Decreased vocal intensity

Objective 3a. Softer voice at the level of words and phrases

Objective 3b. Softer voice at the level of conversational speech

Treatment Procedures

Objectives 1a and 1b. During the first week, the frequency and durations of Roshana's telephone conversations will be baserated. She will be asked to keep a diary to record the number of daily telephone conversations and their durations. During the second week, Roshana will be asked to reduce by 10% the amount of telephone conversation time. She may achieve this by reducing the frequency of telephone conversations or their durations. She will continue to record the frequency and duration of telephone conversations. In subsequent weeks, she will be asked to progressively decrease the amount of time spent on the telephone until the duration is reduced by about 50%.

The frequency of shouting also will be similarly baserated. Roshana will then be asked to reduce the frequency of shouting behavior in 10% decrements until the frequency approaches zero.

Objectives 2a and 2b. The Visi-Pitch will be used to shape a higher pitch consistent with Roshana's gender and age. The treatment will start at the word and phrase level and move on to the conversational speech level.

Objectives 3a and 3b. The Visi-Pitch will be used to progressively decrease the vocal intensity until it is clinically judged to be appropriate for Roshana. The treatment will start at the word and phrase level and move to the conversational speech level.

A maintenance program that includes an analysis of speech samples from home and periodic follow-up and booster treatment will be implemented.

Signed ______________________________
Pero Boss, BA
Student Clinician

I understand the results of the evaluation and agree to the recommended treatment plan.

Signed ______________________________
Roshana Hersh

Signed ______________________________ Date ____________________
Moss Nero, MA, CCC-SLP
Speech-Language Pathologist
Clinical Supervisor

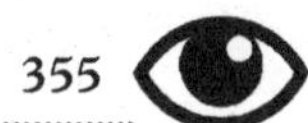

C.7. Practice in Writing Treatment Plans

On the following pages, you will find opportunities to practice writing treatment plans. Clinical data are given on the left-hand page. Use these data to write your treatment plans on the right-hand page.

You may consult the corresponding exemplars in sections C.5 and C.6 before you write the reports in this section. Vary your sentences.

Clinics vary in their format of treatment plans. The format used in this book does not include formally arranged identifying information that was included in assessment (diagnostic reports). However, if required by your clinic, you can place the identifying information at the beginning of the report in the following (or any other accepted) format:

Treatment Plan

Client:	Date of Birth:
Address:	Clinic File Number:
City:	Date:
Telephone Number:	Diagnosis:
Referred By:	Clinician:
Supervisor:	

C.7.1. Practice Writing Comprehensive Treatment Plan: *Child Language Disorder*

University Speech and Hearing Center
Pan Pacific University
Pacifica, California

Data Sheet. Use these data to write your report on the opposite page. Use the correct headings.

Harvey Brokert, 6 years, 5 months

Talks in two- to three-word phrases

No sentences; no bound morphemes

Treatment was recommended

Mother brings the child to treatment

Good prognosis for improved language skills, suggested by good imitation of selected language targets

Final target behaviors: Functional grammatical, syntactic, and pragmatic language skills produced in natural settings

Background Information (L1H)
Who, how old, when, to where referred?
What were the results of evaluation? (Summarize the disorder.)
Was treatment recommended?

Target behaviors? (L1H)

Initial target behaviors: Teaching nouns, auxiliary *is* and verb + *ing*; prepositions *in*, *on*, and *under*; and pronouns *he* and *she*; all taught in the context of simple sentences on discrete trials

Baserated on a set of modeled and evoked trials; 20 stimulus sentences for each target; baserates between 0 and 10%

Write your report. Use the information on the data sheet. Invent information as needed.

Data Sheet. Use these data to write your report on the opposite page. Use the correct headings.

Treatment and probe procedures? (L1H)

Discrete trial procedure:

Show the stimulus, ask a question, model the response, reinforce or give corrective feedback, record the response (correct or incorrect), represent the stimulus for the next trial

Modeling, verbal praise, natural consequences

Five consecutively and correctly imitated responses: shift to evoked trials

Two incorrect responses on evoked trials: reinstate modeling

Various training and probe criteria

Training criterion: Ten consecutively correct, nonimitated responses for each target exemplar (phrase or sentence)

Intermixed probe procedure: Will consist of trained and untrained sentences; trained responses will be reinforced; untrained responses will not be

Correct probe response rate calculated based only on responses given to untrained (probe) stimuli

Ninety percent correct probe response rate: Shift training to another stimulus item, a more complex response topography, or another target behavior.

Probe criterion not met: Give more training on the same target behavior.

Eventually, train the target structures in conversational speech with social reinforcers.

Write your report. Use the information on the data sheet. Invent information as needed.

Data Sheet. Use these data to write your report on the opposite page. Use the correct headings.

Maintenance program (L1H)]

Training family members and others

Teaching the mother to evoke and reinforce the target language structures at home

Initially, the mother observes sessions.

Then she learns to present stimulus items.

Then she learns to reinforce or give corrective feedback.

An older brother to be taught to reinforce target responses

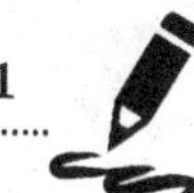

Write your report. Use the information on the data sheet. Invent information as needed.

Data Sheet. Use these data to write your report on the opposite page. Use the correct headings.

Informal training in nonclinical settings (specify a few settings)	Training in informal settings
Recorded home samples for probe analysis; 90% correct production at home is the maintenance criterion.	Home samples
Additional training on other language structures to be determined later	Additional training
	Signature lines
	Student clinician
	Client
	Supervisor

Write your report. Use the information on the data sheet. Invent information as needed.

C.7.2. Practice Writing Brief Treatment Plan: *Stuttering*

Speech and Hearing Clinic
Eastern State University
Bedford, California

Data Sheet. Use these data to write your report on the opposite page. Use the correct headings.

Ezra Bond, 8-year-old boy Parent-referred	Who, how old, when, to where referred?
Two speech samples; dysfluency frequency of 12% and 13% of words spoken in two conversational speech samples (part-word repetitions, sound prolongations, word and phrase interjections, and broken words)	What were the results of evaluation? (Summarize the disorder.)
Treatment was recommended. Prognosis judged to be good because of expressed high parental support for sustained treatment	Was treatment recommended?
Final treatment target: Fluent conversational speech with no more than 5% dysfluency in nonclinical settings Initial targets: Simpler word and phrase utterances, gradually increased to typical sentences	Final treatment objective and the target behaviors? (L1H)

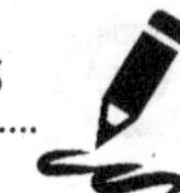

Write your report. Use the information on the data sheet. Invent information as needed.

Data Sheet. Use these data to write your report on the opposite page. Use the correct headings.

Initial baserating in conversational speech

Training to begin with single words and short phrases

Treatment procedure to be used: Response cost. Ezra will be praised and awarded a token for every fluent production (no dysfluencies). Every single dysfluency will result in a token loss with a verbal statement: "Oh, I heard a bump!" The statement may be varied.

All dysfluencies will be counted in all sessions.

Conversational speech with a dysfluency frequency of 2% or less in the clinic will be stabilized across a minimum of three sessions.

Recorded naturalistic conversational probes without treatment to assess generalization

Parent training to verbally reinforce fluency at home

Home speech samples to evaluate maintenance of fluency

A schedule of follow-up; booster treatment

Treatment procedures? (L1H)

Signature lines

Student clinician

Client

Supervisor

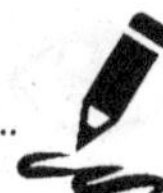

Write your report. Use the information on the data sheet. Invent information as needed.

C.7.3. Practice Writing Brief Treatment Plan: *Speech Sound Disorder*

Valley Speech and Hearing Center
Nordstrom, Maine

Data Sheet. Use these data to write your report on the opposite page. Use the correct headings.

Beth Hazleton, 9 years of age

Speech sound disorder; omissions: (specify four to six phonemes); substitutions: (specify a few)

Treatment recommended

Mother to participate in treatment

Who, how old, when, to where referred? What were the results of evaluation? (Summarize the disorder.) Was treatment recommended?

Ninety percent correct production in conversational speech in extraclinical situations

Final treatment objective? **(Paragraph heading)**

Objective 1. Correct production in all word positions (specify) with 90% accuracy

Procedures: Instructions, demonstrations, modeling, visual feedback, shaping, verbal reinforcement, corrective feedback; discrete trials procedure

All correct and incorrect speech sound productions will be counted.

Objectives? Procedures? **(Paragraph headings)**

Objective 2. Correct production in phrases and sentences

Procedures: Picture description and controlled conversation; modeling, reinforcement, corrective feedback

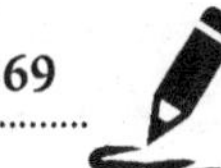

Write your report. Use the information on the data sheet. Invent information as needed.

Data Sheet. Use these data to write your report on the opposite page. Use the correct headings.

Objective 3. Correct production, conversational speech, varied audience

Procedures: Reinforcement, varied audience

Objective 4. Correct production in extraclinical situations

Procedures: Prompting and reinforcing correct production in extraclinical settings (specify)

Objective 5. Teaching the mother (*specify what you teach her*)

Procedures: Initial observation, recognition of the target responses, reinforcement, home treatment sessions, taped home samples to be submitted

Dismissal criterion, follow-up, booster treatment

Paragraph headings for objectives and procedures

Signature lines

Student clinician

Parent

Supervisor

Write your report. Use the information on the data sheet. Invent information as needed.

C.7.4. Practice Writing Brief Treatment Plan: *Child Language Disorder*

Speech and Hearing Clinic
Southern State University
Johnstonville, Louisiana

Data Sheet. Use these data to write your report on the opposite page. Use the correct headings.

Harold Ford, 5 years, 7 months; developmentally delayed Says only six to eight words No phrases, no sentences, no bound morphemes	Who, how old, when, to where referred? What were the results of evaluation? (Summarize the disorder.)
Treatment was recommended	Was treatment recommended?
Correct production of 20 functional words or two-word phrases at 90% accuracy (invent words or phrases) Baserates: 5% to 10% correct	Initial treatment objectives? **Select a heading style**
Additional words Expansion of single words into phrases and sentences Bound morphemes (specify four)	Subsequent treatment objectives? **Repeat the selected heading style**

Write your report. Use the information on the data sheet. Invent information as needed.

Data Sheet. Use these data to write your report on the opposite page. Use the correct headings.

Stimuli to include pictures and so forth (expand)

Clinician and the mother to evoke the target language structures

Initially, approximations accepted; subsequently, more accurate productions required

Verbal praise and natural reinforcers

Measurement of responses in each session

Training criterion: 90% accuracy across two sessions for words; then an intermixed probe to be conducted

Phrases formed out of words that meet the 90% accurate probe criterion

Similar progression for sentences (describe)

Home treatment sessions

Taped home samples to monitor home treatment

Subsequent treatment procedures

The same procedure described under initial treatment procedures Additional words expanded into phrases and sentences

Teaching bound morphemes initially in words, which are later expanded into phrases and sentences

Initial treatment procedures?

Repeat the selected heading style

Subsequent treatment procedures

Repeat the selected heading style

Signature lines

Student clinician

Client

Supervisor

Write your report. Use the information on the data sheet. Invent information as needed.

C.7.5. Practice Writing Brief Treatment Plan: *Voice Disorder*

The Sunshine Speech and Hearing Center
Zanesville, South Dakota

Data Sheet. Use these data to write your report on the opposite page. Use the correct headings.

Thomas Benson, Jr., 28 years of age

Long history of high-pitched voice

Laryngologist has cleared for voice treatment

> Who, how old, when, to where referred?
>
> What were the results of evaluation? (Summarize the disorder.)

Treatment was recommended.

> Was treatment recommended?

Treatment targets

Vocal pitch judged appropriate for age and gender

Lowered pitch level in words, phrases, sentences, and conversational speech (write them as separate goals)

> Use the format given in C.6.4. Brief Treatment Plan: *Voice Disorder*
>
> **Select a heading style and use it consistently**

Write your report. Use the information on the data sheet. Invent information as needed.

Data Sheet. Use these data to write your report on the opposite page. Use the correct headings.

Shaping lower-pitched voice through modeling and verbal feedback

Starting with words and progressing to conversational speech

Other procedures you select

Brief speech sample, recorded periodically, will be used to judge the acceptability of pitch.

Ninety percent accuracy at each level of training

Ninety percent probe criterion in natural settings

Home samples to monitor voice at home

Self-monitoring skills

Teaching Ms. Moline Benson (the client's wife) to monitor and reinforce appropriate pitch at home and to conduct informal home treatment sessions

Home sample to evaluate the home treatment sessions

Standard follow-up and booster treatment

Treatment procedures

Use the selected heading style

Teach family members and others

Signature lines

Student clinician

Supervisor

Client

Write your report. Use the information on the data sheet. Invent information as needed.

Note to Student Clinicians

Clinical supervisors tend to have their preferred formats for writing treatment plans. Talk to your supervisor before you write treatment plans for your clients.

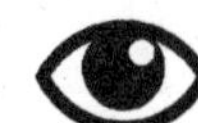

C.8. Progress Reports

Progress reports summarize the methods and results of treatment given during a specified period of time. In academic degree programs, progress reports, also known as *final summaries*, are typically written at the end of a quarter or semester. Schools, hospitals, and private clinics have setting-specific policy and formats. Generally, insurance companies and government or private agencies that pay for services may require monthly progress reports. In all settings, a progress report is written at the time of dismissal from services.

Progress reports that students write under clinical practicum or internship give additional information such as the number and duration of sessions and the clock hours of clinical practicum. Professionals do not include such information.

Most progress reports are formal documents written for the file. Progress reports may be written in the form of a letter to a referring professional or to a funding agency.

Formats used for progress reports vary across clinics. In university clinics, progress reports are written at the end of each quarter or semester. The reports that follow in this section show a few variations. For example, the first report on stuttering refers the reader to a treatment plan in the folder and, therefore, does not summarize the procedures. The next report on a speech disorder makes no mention of a treatment plan; instead, it summarizes the procedures and results (progress).

Progress reports are also written at the end of each treatment session. These session-by-session records include the clinician's subjective evaluation as well as objective data on the target behaviors. Called subjective, objective, assessment, and plan (SOAP), these reports are brief. An example of a SOAP note, written in a medical setting, is provided in C.8.6.

In clinical practicum, students may be required to record the client's response accuracy on treatment trials so that the percent correct response rate may be calculated for each session. A trial-by-trial recording sheet that students may use in clinical practicum is more quantitatively detailed than SOAP notes. An example of a treatment data recording sheet used in each session is provided in C.8.1.

Student clinicians should consult their clinic director or clinical supervisor to find out the format adopted for the clinic or setting.

C.8.1. Trial-by-Trial Data Recording Sheet for Treatment Sessions

Name:	Date: Session #: 4
Age:	Clinician:
Disorder:	Target Behavior:
Criterion:	Reinforcement:

Target Behavior	**Responses on Blocks of 10 Training Trials**									
	1	**2**	**3**	**4**	**5**	**6**	**7**	**8**	**9**	**10**
1.										
Percent correct	Modeled:							Evoked:		
2.										
Percent correct	Modeled:							Evoked:		
3.										
Percent correct	Modeled:							Evoked:		

Target Behavior	Responses on Blocks of 10 Training Trials									
	1	2	3	4	5	6	7	8	9	10
4.										
Percent correct	Modeled:							Evoked:		

Note: This is a progress recording sheet for the *discrete trials* treatment procedure. You may write the following notations in the boxes: + = Correct response; – = Incorrect; 0 = No responses; m = modeled trial; e = Evoked trial (no modeling).

Target behaviors may be correct production of phonemes, grammatical morphemes, fluent utterances, comprehension of sentences, confrontational naming, and so forth.

C.8.2. Progress Report: *Treatment of Stuttering*

University Speech and Hearing Clinic
Freemont University
Valleyville, California

Progress Report

Name: Matt Dexter
Date of Birth: [month, date, year].
Address:
City, State, Zip:
Telephone Number:
Supervisor: Linda Hensley, PhD, CCC-SLP
File Number: Rs92019
Diagnosis: Stuttering
Date of Report: [month, date, year].
Period Covered:
Clinician: Meena Wong

Clinic Schedule

Sessions per week: 3
Length of sessions: 50 min
Number of clinic visits: 24
Clock hr of individual therapy: 25
Clock hr of group therapy: 0
Total clock hr of therapy: 25

Matt Dexter, a 21-year-old male college student, was enrolled for his first semester of treatment for stuttering at the University Speech and Hearing Clinic on February xx, xxxx. An assessment done on [month, date, year] had revealed a 21.2% dysfluency frequency in conversational speech produced in the clinic. It may be rated as a severe stuttering. A home speech sample had revealed a dysfluency rate of 18.6%. He exhibited interjections, pauses, part-word and whole-word repetitions, silent and audible prolongations, pauses, revisions, and incomplete phrases. An assessment report may be found in Mr. Dexter's folder.

Treatment began on [month, date, year].

Summary of Treatment

Final Treatment Objective

Maintenance of fluent conversational speech with a dysfluency frequency of 5% or less in natural settings.

Target Behaviors

Shorter fluent utterances (words and phrases) in the beginning stages. Progressive increases in response complexity. Eventually fluent and naturalistic conversational speech. Please see Mr. Dexter's file for his treatment plan for details.

Treatment Procedures

Dysfluencies were baserated in two clinic samples of conversational speech and a home sample. Mr. Dexter's dysfluency rates were, respectively, 22%, 21%, and 19%.

Treatment procedures included time-out from positive reinforcement (TO) combined with a slight prolongation of initial syllables of the initial words in utterances (phrases or sentences). A slight syllable prolongation of only the initial syllable that did not affect prosody was necessary because of Mr. Dexter's severe stuttering. Syllable prolongation reduced the frequency of dysfluencies on the initial words and allowed for fewer time-out periods.

Instructions were given on syllable prolongation and the time-out procedure. Slight initial syllable prolongation was modeled at the beginning of therapy and whenever judged necessary. Therapy was started at the word level and progressed to phrases, sentences, and conversational speech in the clinic. Corrective feedback was given for a failure to prolong the initial syllables of initial words of utterances. To fluent utterances, the clinician responded typically (eye contact, attention, smile, nod, etc.). At the onset of each dysfluency, the clinician said, "Stop," and terminated eye contact for a period of 5 s (the time-out duration). At the end of the duration, the clinician reestablished the eye contact and said, "please continue." At each level of response complexity, 98% fluency was required.

After Mr. Dexter had progressed to conversational speech, the initial syllable prolongation was gradually faded. He was taught to chart his dysfluencies and failure to prolong the initial syllables. Periodically, Mr. Dexter orally read printed stories and then summarized what he had read. Student observers occasionally participated in treatment sessions to engage in conversation with the client.

Progress

A systematic decrease in the frequency of dysfluencies was recorded in treatment sessions. By mid-semester, his dysfluency frequency in treatment sessions ranged between 6% and 7%. During the 17th treatment session, a 10-min conversational probe was recorded. Mr. Dexter was asked to speak in his typical manner with no syllable prolongation. The time-out contingency was withdrawn. Analysis of the probe data showed 10.5%, compared to 19% to 22% baserate frequency. Treatment was continued without syllable prolongation until the end of the semester (a total of 25 sessions).

A final conversational speech sample containing 852 words in 102 utterances was obtained in the semester's final session. No treatment procedures were in effect. This sample consisted of a conversation with a student observer in the absence of the clinician. Results were as follows:

Dysfluency Types	**Frequency**
Pauses	8
Part-word repetitions	2
Whole-word repetitions	3
Phrase repetitions	2
Sound prolongations	6
Silent prolongations	4
Incomplete phrases	2
Total number of words	**852**
Total dysfluencies	**37**
Percent dysfluency	**5.37**

The results show that Mr. Dexter's fluency improved over the course of the semester. He was about 21% dysfluent at the beginning of treatment compared to 5.37% at the end of the semester.

Recommendations

Time constraints prevented implementation of a generalization and maintenance program. Mr. Dexter's wife and a colleague of his had agreed to participate in treatment sessions to learn ways of supporting his fluency. Therefore, it is recommended that Mr. Dexter continue to receive treatment next semester. The clinician may target the following:

- generalization and maintenance of fluent speech to naturalistic settings
- training his wife and colleague in subtle management of treatment contingencies at home and work situation

Submitted By ______________________________
Layang Chan, BA
Student Clinician

Client's Signature ___________________________ Date: ______________
Mr. Matt Dexter

Approved By ______________________________
Linda Hensley, PhD, CCC-SLP
Speech-Language Pathologist
Clinical Supervisor

C.8.3. Progress Report: *Treatment of Speech Sound Disorder*

Speech and Hearing Center
Henry Higgins Children's Hospital
Burlington, Vermont

Progress Report

Period Covered: xx/xx/xxxx to xx/xx/xxxx

Background Information

Joe Villa, a 6-year and 3-month-old boy, was seen for a speech and language evaluation at the Speech and Hearing Center of the Henry Higgins Children's Hospital on September xx, xxxx. Joe has an articulation disorder characterized mostly by omissions of /s/, /t/, /k/, /b/, and /l/ in the initial and final positions of words. An articulation treatment program was recommended. He has received treatment at this facility for 4 months.

The final treatment objective for Joe was to produce the phonemes he omits with 90% accuracy in conversational speech in extraclinical situations.

Progress

Objective 1. Correct production of /s/, /t/, /k/, /b/, and /l/ in word initial position with 90% accuracy

Method and Results: The target phoneme production in word initial positions was baserated on a set of modeled and evoked trials with 20 words for each phoneme. Joe's correct response rate ranged from 0 to 10%. Treatment was begun with the discrete trial procedure involving modeling, imitation, successive approximation, and immediate verbal feedback for correct and incorrect responses. Whenever necessary, the tongue positions were shown with the help of a mirror. Each target sound was trained to a criterion of 10 consecutively correct responses. When four words with a target sound met the training criterion, at least 10 probe words were presented to assess generalization.

Joe has met this training objective. His correct response rates on these phonemes in word initial positions varied between 95% and 100%.

Objective 2. Correct production of /s/, /t/, /k/, /b/, and /l/ in word final position with 90% accuracy

Methods and Results: The same procedures used to train the phonemes in the word initial position were used. Joe has met this objective. His correct response rates on the phonemes in word final position varied between 92% and 96%.

Objective 3. Production of the target sounds in phrases and sentences with 90% accuracy in all word positions

Method and Results: Joe's correct productions were initially reinforced in phrases that were prepared for training. Soon, he was asked to use the target words in sentences he formulated. Later, Joe's conversational speech was monitored to strengthen the correct production of the phonemes. Verbal reinforcement was used on an FR4 schedule.

Joe has met this objective as his correct production of the target phonemes in conversational speech varied between 90% and 95%.

Objective 4. The development and implementation of a home program to maintain the production of his new speech skills in natural settings with 90% accuracy

Methods and Results: Joe's parents, who attended most of the treatment sessions, were taught to recognize, prompt, and reinforce the correct production of target sounds. His parents were asked to hold home treatment sessions twice a week and to tape-record the sessions. These taped samples were analyzed to give feedback to the parents. Three conversational probes recorded at home have revealed a 90% correct response rate.

Overall, Joe has made excellent progress in producing the targeted sounds. All treatment objectives have been met. Therefore, it is recommended that Joe be dismissed from treatment. A follow-up assessment in 3 months is recommended.

Signed By ______________________________

Monica Mendoza, MA, CCC-SLP
Speech-Language Pathologist

 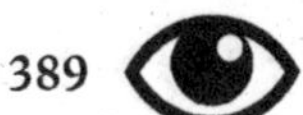

C.8.4. Progress Report: *Treatment of Child Language Disorder*

University Speech and Hearing Center
Bellview University
Bellview, Washington

Progress Report

Client: William Shakespeare
Date of Birth: January xx, xxxx
Period Covered: xx/xx through xx/xx, xxxx
Clinician: Noah Webster

Clinic Schedule

Sessions per week: 2
Length of sessions: 40 min
Number of clinic visits: 24
Clock hr of individual therapy: 25
Clock hr of group therapy: 0
Total clock hr of therapy: 25

William Shakespeare, a 7-year, 3-month-old boy, was assessed for a language disorder at the University Speech and Hearing Center of Bellview University. The assessment suggested that his language disorder primarily involved some syntactic structures and pragmatic functions. Treatment was recommended. He has received treatment for one semester. Please see his clinic file for an assessment report and a complete treatment program.

Summary of Treatment

William was cooperative in most treatment sessions. The following treatment procedures and objectives were used.

Objective 1. Asking* wh *questions

William was taught to ask the following types of *wh* questions:

- What do you mean?
- What is it?
- What are you doing?
- What time is it?
- What is your name?

Methods and Results: Baserating showed that William typically did not ask the target questions even when the situation demanded them. In a conversational role-playing situation, William was taught to ask the target questions. Conversational situations were created such that questions of the kind targeted would be appropriate. Conversation was manipulated in various ways to prompt the target question. For example, William was asked, "Do you live in a condo?" and the correct question was immediately modeled for him to imitate: "William, ask me *what do you mean*?" Or he was shown a picture he did not know anything about and immediately the question "What is it?" was modeled for him to imitate. When William imitated modeled questions or asked similar questions without modeling, the clinician correctly answered them. These answers and verbal praise for asking appropriate questions were the reinforcers.

When William's question-asking reached 90% accuracy, probes were conducted to assess generalized question-asking. The probe results showed that William learned to ask the targeted questions in untrained (probe) contexts with 90% accuracy.

Objective 2. Topic Maintenance

William was taught to maintain a topic of conversation for progressively increasing durations with 90% accuracy.

Methods and Results: Baserating showed that William typically changed the topic in less than a minute. He was taught to maintain a topic of conversation for progressively longer durations. One-minute increments were used. Starting with a duration of 1 min, he was taught to talk about the same topic for a maximum duration of 5 min. Every time he deviated from the topic, the clinician asked him to stop and prompted him to resume the target topic. He was periodically praised for continuing on the same topic.

William learned to maintain a topic of conversation for a minimum of 5 min. On certain probe topics, he continued to talk for up to 10 min.

Objective 3. Conversational turn taking

William was taught to take appropriate conversational turns with 90% accuracy.

Methods and Results: During the baserating, William typically interrupted the clinician every 30 s. He was initially asked to speak only when told, "It is your turn to talk." The clinician gave William his turn every minute or so. William also was taught to say, "It is your turn to talk" when he had spoken for a minute or so. If he did not, he was asked to stop at the end of a sentence. The prompt, "It is your turn to talk," was withdrawn in the later training sessions. If he interrupted, the clinician gave a hand signal to stop. This signal also was faded. In the last four sessions, a variable time interval of 1–3 min of talking before yielding the floor was allowed.

William learned to take conversational turns. On a final probe with no verbal or manual prompt, he took turns on the variable time schedule of 1–3 min of talking with 90% accuracy. Occasionally, he appropriately exceeded the range.

A final spontaneous language sample was analyzed to determine the need for further clinical services. The analysis revealed normal language use. Therefore, it is recommended that William be dismissed from treatment.

Signed By ______________________________

Noah Webster, BA
Student Clinician

Mother's Signature ______________________________

Mrs. Tara Shakespeare

Signed By ______________________________

Lakshmi Shanker, PhD, CCC-SLP
Speech-Language Pathologist and Clinical Supervisor

C.8.5. Progress Report: *Treatment of Voice Disorder*

Sunshine Speech and Hearing Center
Kingsville, Vermont

Progress Report

Name: Roshana Hersh

Date of Birth: xx-xx-xxxx

Address: 7915 Vishon

City: Clovis, CA 93611

Telephone Number: (xxx) xxx-xxxx

Supervisor: Moss Nero, MA, CCC-SLP

File Number: Ax1cq12-3

Diagnosis: Voice Disorder

Date of Report: xx-xx-xxxx

Period Covered: [xx-xx-xxxx to xx-xx-xxxx

Clinician: Pero Boss

Roshana Hersh, a 21-year-old female college student, was seen at the Sunshine Speech and Hearing Center on March xx, xxxx, for a voice evaluation. The evaluation suggested a pattern of vocal abuse associated with a persistent hoarseness of voice and low pitch. A treatment program to improve her voice quality was recommended. The assessment report and a description of her treatment program may be found in her clinical file.

Treatment Targets

Goal 1:

Production of clear voice at least 90% of the time Ms. Hersh speaks by reducing the hoarseness of voice

Objective 1a. Reduced amount of talking over the phone

Objective 1b. Reduced amount of shouting at school

Goal 2:

Increased vocal pitch

Objective 2a. Higher pitch at the level of words and phrases

Objective 2b. Higher pitch at the level of conversational speech

Treatment Procedures and Results

Objectives 1a and 1b

During the first week, the durations of Ms. Hersh's telephone conversation were baserated. The diary record she kept showed that Roshana spoke between 8 and 10 times over the phone each day and that the duration of her phone calls ranged from 10 to 20 min. Sixty percent of her phone calls typically exceeded 15 min.

During the second week, Ms. Hersh was asked to reduce by 10% the amount of telephone conversation time. She continued to record the amount of time she spent talking over the phone. In subsequent weeks, she was asked to progressively decrease the amount of time spent on the telephone with a goal of reducing the duration by about 50%.

The frequency of shouting also was similarly baserated. On an average day, she tended to shout 8 to 10 times. Ms. Hersh was asked to reduce the frequency of shouting behavior in 10% decrements until the frequency approached zero.

Ms. Hersh made excellent progress in reducing the frequency and duration of phone calls and in reducing the frequency of shouting. At the end of the semester, her phone calls averaged from 3 to 7 min. Only an occasional phone call exceeded this range. Her shouting behavior was reduced to no more than two incidents per day. According to Ms. Hersh, her shouts are not as loud as they used to be.

Objectives 2a and 2b

The Visi-Pitch was used to shape a higher pitch consistent with Ms. Hersh's gender and age. The treatment was started at the word and phrase level and moved to the conversational speech level.

Ms. Hersh's speaking fundamental frequency in the clinic increased from a baserate of 157 Hz to 200 Hz toward the end of the semester. However, she still reports a much lower pitch outside the clinic.

It is recommended that Ms. Hersh continue to receive voice therapy next semester. The emphasis should be on generalization and maintenance of appropriate target vocal characteristics in extraclinical situations. Ms. Hersh needs training in self-monitoring skills.

Signed By ______________________________

Pero Boss, BA
Student Clinician

Client's Signature ______________________________

Ms. Roshana Hersh

Signed By ______________________________ Date ________________

Moss Nero, MA, CCC-SP
Speech-Language Pathologist
Clinical Supervisor

C.8.6. SOAP Progress Report

Sierra View Hospital
Nugget, Mississippi

Name of Patient: Date of Birth:

File #: Clinician(s):

Date and Initials	Progress Note
1-5-23 KPS	Ms. Muelenhouser looked tired this morning. She smiled at me but did not respond when I said, "Good morning!" She said, "I didn't sleep well last night." Her answers to 10 questions about time, place, and the names of attending staff were 60% correct. In a short story retelling, she produced seven grammatically complete sentences out of 10 (70% accuracy). In a 30-min individual therapy session, Ms. Muelenhouser named objects with 60% accuracy (40% during in the previous session). She maintained conversation on the same topic for 4 min (2 min during the previous session). Ms. Muelenhouser is showing consistent improvement across sessions. The same treatment on the same targets will be continued.
1-15-23 KPS	Ms. Muelenhouser was alert and cheerful this morning. Said, "Good morning" upon seeing me. In a short story retell, she produced 10 grammatically complete sentences out of 10 (100% accuracy, the same during the previous two sessions). In a 30-min individual therapy session, Ms. Muelenhouser named objects with 95% accuracy (the same during the previous two sessions). She maintained conversation on the same topic for 6 min (the same during the previous two sessions). Ms. Muelenhouser has met the training criteria for grammaticality, naming, and conversational topic maintenance. Topic initiation and conversational repair will be the new treatment targets beginning with the next session. The same treatment procedure will be used.

Note: The first paragraph in each box is a *subjective* statement (clinician's impressions). The last two paragraphs are *analysis* and the *plan* for the next session. The paragraphs in between give *objective* data on target behaviors. Notice the change in treatment plan in the entry for 1-15-23.

Note to Student Clinicians

Contact your clinic director to find out how progress reports vary in your clinic. Contact a private speech and hearing clinic and a speech-language pathology department in your area hospital to find out how clinicians there write progress reports they send to health insurance companies.

C.9. Practice in Writing Progress Reports

This section provides treatment progress data on the left-hand pages and right-hand blank pages to practice writing progress reports. During clinical practicum in university clinics, students are likely to write progress reports similar to the template given in this section.

Practice formats are provided for stuttering in an adult, speech sound disorder in a child, language disorder in a child, and voice disorder in an adult.

C.9.1. Practice Writing Progress Report: *Treatment of Stuttering*

University Speech and Hearing Clinic
Freemont University
Valleyville, California

Progress Report

Name: Winston Churchill	File Number:
Date of Birth:	Diagnosis: Stuttering
Address:	Date of Report:
City:	Period Covered:
Telephone Number:	Clinician:

Clinic Schedule

Sessions per week:	Clock hr of individual therapy:
Length of sessions:	Clock hr of group therapy:
Number of clinic visits:	Total clock hr of therapy:

Data Sheet. Use these data to write your report on the opposite page. Use the correct headings.

Winston Churchill, 22 years of age; college student.

Who, how old, came to which clinic, and with what problem?

Stuttering since early childhood days; various ineffective treatments in the past

Two conversational speech samples showed dysfluency frequencies of 9% and 11% of words spoken

One reading sample (15% dysfluency)

(Summarize the assessment data in one or two sentences.)

Received treatment for stuttering for one semester at the same facility; the same treatment as described next

Received treatment for what and for how long?

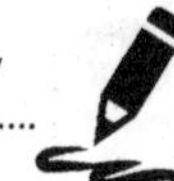

Write your report. Use the information on the data sheet. Invent information as needed.

Data Sheet. Use these data to write your report on the opposite page. Use the correct headings.

Select a heading style and use it consistently.

Baselines

Treatment targets

Treatment, probe, and measurement procedures

Final treatment goal: Fluent speech in natural settings with a dysfluency frequency that is less than 5% of words spoken (or any other objectives your supervisor suggests)

Two conversational speech baserates of 10% and 11% dysfluency (or stuttering); based on the number of words spoken

Treatment target: Reduction in dysfluencies in treatment sessions and nonclinical settings including home and college

Treatment procedure: Time-out from positive reinforcement. Termination of social reinforcers that accompany typical conversation for a brief duration of 5 s contingent on each dysfluency. Conversation in all sessions.

At the onset of each dysfluency, the clinician said, "Stop," and avoided eye contact. Mr. Churchill remained silent for the duration. At the end of the duration, the clinician reestablished eye contact and asked him to "Continue."

Periodic probes with no treatment contingencies to assess generalized fluency; thrice-a-week sessions of 50 min; dysfluencies measured in all sessions.

Roommate taught to prompt and reinforce fluent speech in brief conversations.

Write your report. Use the information on the data sheet. Invent information as needed.

Data Sheet. Use these data to write your report on the opposite page. Use the correct headings.

Results or Progress

Good progress: Dysfluency frequency reduced to 5% in conversational probes in the clinic (two probe conversational speech samples), 7% at home (one home speech sample)

Continued treatment recommended to further reduce the dysfluencies and to stabilize fluency in naturalistic settings through informal treatment in various nonclinical settings (specify a few)

Your name, degree, and title

Client's name

Your supervisor's name, degree, certification, and title

Continue with the selected heading style

What were the results? Recommendations

Signature lines

Student clinician

Client

Supervisor

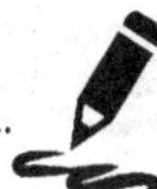

Write your report. Use the information on the data sheet. Invent information as needed.

C.9.2. Practice Writing Progress Report: *Treatment of Speech Sound Disorder*

University Speech and Hearing Center
Bloom, Illinois

Progress Report

Name: Jimmy Jones	File Number:
Date of Birth:	Diagnosis: Speech Sound Disorder
Address:	Date of Report:
City:	Period Covered:
Telephone Number:	Clinician:

Clinic Schedule

Sessions per week:	Clock hr of individual therapy:
Length of sessions:	Clock hr of group therapy:
Number of clinic visits:	Total clock hr of therapy:

Data Sheet. Use these data to write your report on the opposite page. Use the correct headings.

Jimmy Jones, 6 years, 7 months

Who, how old, came to which clinic, and with what problem?

Speech sound disorder

Omissions of initial and final /k, s, t, p, b/

(Summarize the assessment data in one or two sentences.)

No prior treatment

Received treatment for what and for how long?

Write your report. Use the information on the data sheet. Invent information as needed.

Data Sheet. Use these data to write your report on the opposite page. Use the correct headings.

Continue with the selected heading style

Progress or Methods and Results

Treatment objective 1: Teaching the phonemes in word initial and final positions

Baserated: 0 to 5% correct response rate on evoked; 5% to 10% correct response rate on modeled trials

Treatment procedures: Modeling, imitation, successive approximation, visual feedback (phonetic placement); positive reinforcement for correct responses and corrective feedback for wrong responses

Training criterion: Ninety percent correct for any phoneme in any position

Probe criterion: Ninety-five percent correct (intermixed probe: trained and untrained words; reinforcement only for the trained words)

Met the probe criterion for initial and final positions

Production of phonemes in phrases and sentences

Probe: Ninety-five percent correct

Treatment objective 2: Production of target phonemes in phrases and sentences

The same training and probe criteria (specify)

Met the probe criterion for phrases and sentences

Treatment objective 3: Production of target phonemes in conversational speech

The same training and probe criteria (specify)

Did not meet the probe criterion (showed only 70% correct in conversational speech)

Write your report. Use the information on the data sheet. Invent information as needed.

Data Sheet. Use these data to write your report on the opposite page. Use the correct headings.

Continue with the selected heading style

Data	Heading
Development of a home treatment program for maintenance	Maintenance program
Teaching the father to evoke and reinforce the phonemes in conversational speech at home	
Additional treatment to obtain and stabilize correct productions in conversational speech at 90% accuracy	Recommendations
	Signature lines
Your name, degree, and title	Student clinician
The client's father's name	Parent
Your supervisor's name, degree, certification, and title	Supervisor

Write your report. Use the information on the data sheet. Invent information as needed.

C.9.3. Practice Writing Progress Report: *Treatment of Child Language Disorder*

University Speech and Hearing Center Bellview University
Bellview, Washington

Progress Report

Name: Tanya Tucker

File Number:

Date of Birth:

Diagnosis: Language Disorder

Address:

Date of Report:

City:

Period Covered:

Telephone Number:

Clinician:

Clinic Schedule

Sessions per week:

Clock hr of individual therapy:

Length of sessions:

Clock hr of group therapy:

Number of clinic visits:

Total clock hr of therapy:

Data Sheet. Use these data to write your report on the opposite page. Use the correct headings.

Tanya Tucker, 6 years and 8 months

Language disorders. Does not produce *ing*, auxiliary *is*, regular and irregular plurals, regular past tense, prepositions, and pronouns

Two semesters of treatment on teaching functional words and expansion of words into phrases; has met most probe criteria on these

Select a heading style and use it consistently

Who, how old, came to which clinic, and with what problem?

Summarize the assessment data in one or two sentences.

Received treatment for what and for how long?

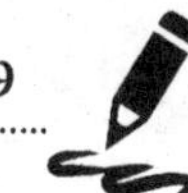

Write your report. Use the information on the data sheet. Invent information as needed.

Data Sheet. Use these data to write your report on the opposite page. Use the correct headings.

Use the selected heading style consistently

Treatment targets: Present progressive *ing*, auxiliary *is*, and regular plural morpheme *s* (e.g., *books* and *cups*) in sentences during the current semester of treatment

Pictures to evoke the target structures

Training criterion: Ninety percent correct in words, phrases, and sentences

Probe criterion: Ninety percent correct on a set of 10 untrained words, and untrained words used in phrases and sentences

Twenty words, phrases, and sentences for each target. Baserate: 0 to 10% correct

Discrete trial training at the level of words, phrases, and sentences

Treatment procedures included stimulus presentation, appropriate question asking, modeling, reinforcement, and corrective feedback

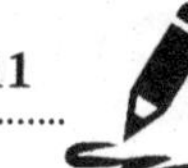

Write your report. Use the information on the data sheet. Invent information as needed.

Data Sheet. Use these data to write your report on the opposite page. Use the correct headings.

Results or Progress

Tanya made good progress in learning the language structures. Met the probe criteria for words and phrases for all targets.

For sentences: Present progressive *ing*: Eight sentences trained; probe response rate: 90% correct probe response rate (thus has met the probe criterion)

Auxiliary *is*: Six sentences trained; 70% correct probe response rate

Regular plural *s* morpheme: four sentences trained; 80% correct probe response rate

Mother has received training in evoking and reinforcing the target structures at home.

A home sample showed: 87% correct for the *ing*; 65% for the auxiliary *is*; and 70% for the plural *s*

Recommendations:

Continued treatment on the auxiliary and the plural morpheme to meet the probe criterion

Training to be shifted to conversational speech level for the present progressive *ing*

Training on additional grammatical morphemes Tanya does not produce

Continue to promote home training

Your name, degree, and title

Parent's name

Your supervisor's name, degree, certification, and title

Use the selected heading style consistently

Signature lines

Student clinician

Parent

Supervisor

Write your report. Use the information on the data sheet. Invent information as needed.

C.9.4. Practice Writing Progress Report: *Treatment of Voice Disorder*

The Sunshine Speech and Hearing Center
Zingsville, Vermont

Progress Report

Name: Raj Mohan	File Number:
Date of Birth:	Diagnosis: Voice Disorder
Address:	Date of Report:
City:	Period Covered:
Telephone Number:	Clinician:

Clinic Schedule

Sessions per week:	Clock hr of individual therapy:
Length of sessions:	Clock hr of group therapy:
Number of clinic visits:	Total clock hr of therapy:

Data Sheet. Use these data to write your report on the opposite page. Use the correct headings.

Select a heading style and use it consistently

Raj Mohan, 35 years of age

High school teacher

Inadequate loudness; voice too soft; students complain; his voice gets tired; ENT report negative; no contraindications for voice therapy

No prior treatment

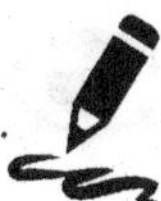

Write your report. Use the information on the data sheet. Invent information as needed.

Data Sheet. Use these data to write your report on the opposite page. Use the correct headings.

Use the selected heading style consistently

Treatment targets:

Increased vocal loudness; adequate loudness for classroom teaching as rated by the clinician and his students across a minimum of four teaching sessions

Baseline of loudness established by: The clinician's and students' rating of loudness on a 5-point rating scale in three class periods

Recording the frequency of student requests for louder speech (invent baseline data)

Treatment procedures

Included verbal reinforcement of progressively louder speech

Masking noise to increase vocal intensity (Lombard effect)

Visi-Pitch feedback to shape progressively louder voice

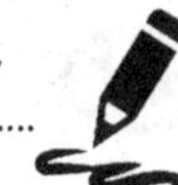

Write your report. Use the information on the data sheet. Invent information as needed.

Data Sheet. Use these data to write your report on the opposite page. Use the correct headings.

Use the selected heading style consistently

Results or Progress

Excellent progress; clinician's rating of loudness in three class periods showed adequate loudness; no student requests for louder speech in the three observed class periods (compare this to baseline data)

Schedule a follow-up in 3 months to assess maintenance of adequate loudness

Recommendations: Dismissal from treatment; 3- and 6-month follow-up and booster treatment if necessary

Your name, degree, and title — Student clinician

Client's name — Client

Supervisor's name, degree, certification, and title — Supervisor

Write your report. Use the information on the data sheet. Invent information as needed.

Note to Student Clinicians

Obtain samples of progress reports from your clinic director. Practice writing reports on other disorders of communication.

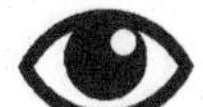

C.10. Report Writing in Public Schools

Speech and language services in public schools are regulated by the state education laws and the policies school districts adopt. Speech-language pathologists (SLPs) in public schools write a variety of reports, some of which are unique to their setting:

- **Assessment reports.** These are similar to diagnostic reports written in other settings but with several special considerations. There is an *initial report* that determines whether the child qualifies for clinical (or special educational) services according to the state laws and the policies of the school district. If the child is enrolled in speech and language services, there may be an annual, biannual, or triannual report to help make decisions regarding the student's promotion to higher grade or transition to regular classroom from special education. Policies on such reports and their frequency may vary from district to district. A sample form of initial assessment that determines whether the child qualifies for speech-language services is provided in C.10.1. The same format may be used for the initial and subsequent assessment reports. Please note that assessment report formats and service eligibility criteria vary across states and school districts within states.
- **Individualized education programs (IEPs).** These are similar to brief treatment plans written in other settings but with some unique features. Several exemplars are provided.
- **Individualized family service plans (IFSPs).** An extended report that includes service offered to the student and family. These are less commonly written in the schools, and therefore, a sample is not provided in this section. For a description of IFSPs, see Hegde and Kuyumjian (2020).
- **SOAP (subjective, objective, assessment, plan).** These are very brief progress notes on individual treatment sessions, written more commonly in medical settings and less commonly in educational settings. An exemplar is provided.

With their heavy caseloads, SLPs in public schools often do not have time to write lengthy or narrative treatment plans for the children they serve. Therefore, they may use several kinds of printed forms to select treatment targets and report progress. Formats vary across school districts, some being more detailed than others. This section provides a few examples of reports clinicians typically write in public schools.

Student clinicians assigned to clinical practicum in a public school should contact the supervising speech-language pathologist at the school at the earliest opportunity to get familiarized with the assessment, treatment, progress, and other kinds of reports they will be expected to write there.

C.10.1. Assessment Report Format

Glacier Point Unified School District
Glacier, Alabama

Speech and Language Evaluation and Service Eligibility

Name:	Date of Birth:	Age:	Grade:
School:	Case Manager:	Evaluator:	Date:

Assessment Information

Informal Measures Used (Check all that apply):

☐ Parent Interview	☐ Teacher Interview	☐ Student interview
☐ Orofacial examination	☐ Spontaneous speech and language sample	
☐ Voice and fluency	☐ Educational observations	☐ Other (specify):

Standardized Tests (specify):

1. ______________________ 2. ______________________ 3. ______________________

4. ______________________ 5. ______________________ 6. ______________________

History and Interview Data

History

Health, Social, Developmental History:

Educational History:

Services Received:

Previous Assessment Results:

Prior Intervention:

Summary of Parent Interview:

Summary of Student Interview:

Summary of Teacher Interview:

Assessment

Information in this report was compiled from multiple sources including informant interviews, review of records, observation of the student, analysis of speech-language behaviors, direct assessment using formal standardized measures, and informal speech/language tasks.

The student was compliant, attentive, and cooperative during multiple assessment sessions. The student answered all questions and completed all assessment tasks. The student's primary language was reported to be English, and therefore, all testing was completed in English. It is judged that the results are representative of the skills tested.

Speech Production and Intelligibility

Oral-Peripheral Examination

Voice and Fluency

Speech Production Assessment(s)

Summarize the results of:

Standardized Tests

Analysis of Speech Sample

Stimulability Testing

Language Production and Comprehension

Summarize the results of:

Standardized Tests Administered

Alternative Assessment Tools [if used]

Analysis of Language Sample

Educational Observations

Summarize the results of the teacher's observation of communication and SLP's in-class observation of the student's speech, language, voice, and fluency skills. Specify whose observation was recorded (teacher or the SLP).

Observation #1: Date

Observation #2: Date

Observation #3: Date

Assessment Instruments and Procedures

Statement on the assessment instruments used: *The assessment materials and procedures used are consistent with the federal and state education codes and the Glacier Point Unified School District policies. All test materials were administered in the pupil's primary language or through the use of an interpreter. All test materials have been validated for the specific purpose for which they are used and were administered by trained personnel following the instructional manuals. Selected assessment materials did not discriminate on the basis of sex, sexual orientation, gender, gender identity, race, or ethnicity.*

Summary and Eligibility

In my opinion, this is a valid assessment of [student's name] speech and language skills and how those skills relate to the student's educational needs.

In program planning and placement considerations for this student, the special education team will review the information obtained in the evaluation, along with other pertinent information from home, school, and other appropriate sources. It is the responsibility of the Special Education team to suggest an appropriate placement for this student in the least restrictive environment.

The student has a language or speech disorder as defined in Education Code ______ section ______, and it is determined that the pupil's disorder meets one or more of the following criteria for a communication disorder:

A. **Articulation Disorder** (check what applies).

- ☐ *The student is eligible for speech and language services.* The student demonstrated consistent errors of two phonemes that were not developmentally appropriate for the student's age. The student's speech intelligibility is low, causing significant difficulty in understanding [the student's] speech. This difficulty is likely to adversely affect educational performance.
- ☐ *The student is not eligible for speech and language services.* The student does not meet the criteria for an articulation disorder because [the student's] communication disability is limited to an abnormal swallowing pattern and inconsistent distortion of a single phoneme that may not adversely affect speech intelligibility or educational performance. The student's speech intelligibility is at least 95%.

B. **Voice disorder**

- ☐ *The student is eligible for speech and language services.* The student has a voice disorder that is characterized by persistently impaired voice quality, pitch, or loudness, affecting everyday communication.
- ☐ *The student is not eligible for speech and language services.* The student's vocal quality, pitch, and loudness were within normal limits for gender and age.

C. **Fluency Disorder**

- ☐ *The student is eligible for speech and language services.* The student has a fluency disorder because the dysfluency rate in conversational speech exceeds 5% of the words spoken.
- ☐ *The student is not eligible for speech and language services.* The student's fluency is within normal limits because the dysfluency rate in conversation was under 5% of the words spoken.

D. **Language Disorder**

- ☐ *The student is eligible for speech and language services.* The student has an expressive or receptive language disorder that is likely to negatively affect the student's educational performance. The student scored 1.5 standard deviations below the mean on [specify two or more tests]. The student scored below the seventh percentile on [specify two or more tests]. The student's performance falls below the norm for the student's chronological age on at least one measure of morphological, syntactic, semantic, or pragmatic skills. A conversational speech sample of 50 utterances revealed deficient or inappropriate production of language structures. [State the names of alternative assessment tools used when standardized tests were considered inappropriate for the student.]
- ☐ *The student is not eligible for speech and language services.* The student's performance did not fall below the seventh percentile on any language measure and did not exhibit inappropriate or deficient production of any of the language structures in a spontaneous language sample.

Respectfully submitted,

____

SLP Name, MA, CCC-SLP
Language Speech Specialist
________ School
________ School District

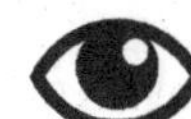

C.10.2. IEP: Treatment of Child Language Disorder

Central Coast Unified School District
Individualized Educational Program for Speech and Language Services
Oral Language and Verbal Expression

Student's Name ______________________ Date of Birth ______________

School ______________________ Grade __________ Date ______________

Speech-Language Pathologist ______________________________

Criteria for Placement ______________________________

Goal: To improve oral language and verbal expression

Present Level of Performance: ***See assessment report***	**Target Date**	**Met On (Date)**	**Not Met**
Objectives: By x/xx [specify the date] the student will complete the following objectives with 90% accuracy as measured by pre- and posttests, specialist's observations, client-specific procedures, or other procedures (specify):	[Specify]		
Improve oral language through:			
Social interaction with others: (Check the targets selected)			
1. ✓ verbally respond when spoken to 2. ✓ verbally express feelings and needs 3. ✓ give personal information upon request 4. ✓ ask and answer questions 5. ✓ initiate conversation 6. ✓ share personal experiences 7. ✓ describe events in detail 8. ✓ report factual information 9. ✓ interact verbally with others 10. ✓ give sequential, accurate verbal directions 11. ✓ take part in class discussions and reports 12. ✓ other ______________	[Specify]		

C.10.3. IEP: Treatment of Speech Sound Disorder

Atlantic Unified School District
Language, Speech, and Hearing
Individualized Educational Program Objectives
Treatment of Speech Sound Disorder

Pupil ______________________________

Speech, Language, and Hearing Specialist ______________________________ Date __________________

School ____ Services started on __________________

Goal: Improved intelligibility of speech through correct production of phonemes at 90% accuracy.

Target Date	Objectives (Check the Ones Selected)	Evaluation and Treatment Procedures	Date Objectives Met
	Speech Sound Production		

[Specify]	Correct production of the following phonemes:
	
	/d/, /t/, /p/, /z/, and /l/
	
	✓ in isolation
	✓ in syllables
	✓ in words
	  ✓ initial
	  ✓ medial
	  ✓ final
	✓ in phrases
	✓ in sentences
	✓ conversational speech
	✓ in natural settings
	
	increased intelligibility
		Paired stimuli method of treatment
		
		Probes to assess production in untrained contexts
			[Specify]

C.10.4. IEP: Treatment of Voice Disorder

Gulf Coast Unified School District
Department of Special Educational Services
Language, Speech, and Hearing
Individualized Educational Program
Treatment of Voice Disorders

Student's Name ______________________________

Speech, Language, and Hearing Specialist ______________________________

School ______________________________

Program Initiation Date ____________________ Date ____________________

Goal: By *x/xx* [specify the date], the student will complete the following objectives with 80% accuracy.

Target Date	Objectives (Check the Ones Selected)	Evaluation and Treatment Procedures	Target Met On (Date)
	Voice Overall objective: Improved voice quality and appropriate use of voice		
[Specify]	**Pitch** ✓ lower __ higher __ in school __ in other settings **Intensity** __ lower (softer voice) ✓ higher (louder voice) __ in school __ in other settings **Nasal resonance** __ decrease __ increase **Voice quality** ✓ reduce hoarseness ✓ reduce harshness ✓ reduce breathiness Other voice objectives (specify):	Successive approximation with the help of Visi-Pitch Conversational probes to assess generalization and maintenance	[Specify]

C.10.5. IEP: Treatment of Stuttering

North Central Unified School District
Speech, Language, and Hearing Services
Individualized Educational Program
Treatment of Stuttering

Student's Name ______________________________ Age ________ Grade ________

Speech, Language, and Hearing Specialist ______________________________

School ______________________________

Treatment Began On ____________________ Date ____________________

Goal: Improved fluency in conversational speech produced in extraclinical settings with a dysfluency rate under 5%.

Target Date	Objectives (Check the Ones Selected)	Evaluation and Treatment Procedures	Objectives Met On
	FLUENCY		
[Specify]	Target skills: ✓ Fluent conversational speech with dysfluencies less than 5% of the words spoken in natural settings ✓Dysfluencies less than 2% of the words spoken in the clinical setting ✓Parental reinforcement of fluent utterances at home	Baselines of fluent utterances and the percentage of dysfluencies will be established in conversational speech. During training, all fluent utterances will be reinforced with verbal praise. Initial targets may be fluently spoken words or phrases. All dysfluencies will be ignored; no corrective feedback will be provided. Parents will be trained to reinforce fluent utterances at home. Periodic conversational speech probes will help assess generalization and maintenance of fluency in clinical and extraclinical settings.	[Specify]

C.10.6. SOAP Note Format

Northwestern Unified School District
Speech, Language, and Hearing Services

SOAP Note

El Capitan Elementary School
El Capitan, Nebraska

Name: Grade:

Date: Minutes/Service: Time:

Session Type: _________ Individual _________ Group

Clinician:

Subjective Impressions:

____ On task/good participation ____ Difficulty attending

____ Positive mood ____ Appeared tired

____ Other ____ Other

Objective Results: Correct production of /s/ in words

	Session date															%
Trials																

	Session date															%
Trials																

	Session date															%
Trials																

Analysis:	
Plan for Next Session:	
_______ Continue treatment	_______ Change stimuli
_______ Increase response complexity	_______ Change setting
Other treatment modifications (specify):	
Signature: Speech-Language Pathologist	

Note: Record the child's response on each trial in one of the boxes. Place a check mark for a correct response, and an *x* for an incorrect response. Calculate the percent correct response rate and enter it under the % column.

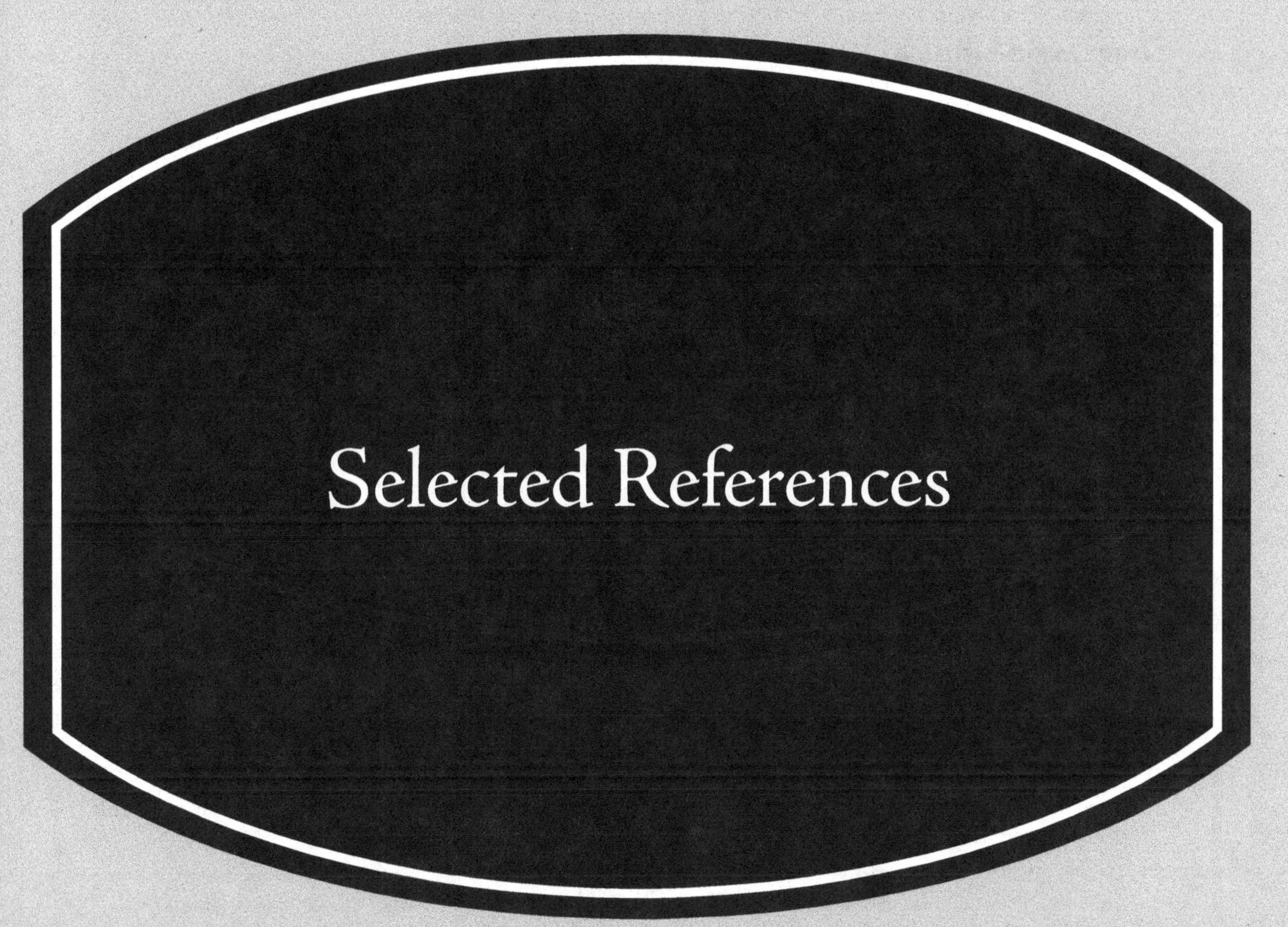

Selected References

Sources on Clinical Report Writing

The clinical assessment, treatment, and progress reports outlined in this coursebook are based on information presented in the textbooks listed here. If you are not sure of clinical terms, assessment techniques, or treatment procedures, consult the following sources. You also may use textbooks you used in courses on clinical methods, including diagnostic procedures. Ask your clinic director, clinic supervisors, or course instructors to recommend other sources.

Hegde, M. N. (2018). *Hegde's PocketGuide to assessment in speech-language pathology* (4th ed.). Plural Publishing.

Hegde, M. N. (2018). *Hegde's PocketGuide to treatment in speech-language pathology* (4th ed.). Plural Publishing.

Hegde, M. N., & Freed, F. (2022). *Assessment of communication disorders in adults* (3rd ed.). Plural Publishing.

Hegde, M. N., & Kuyumjian, K. (2020). *Clinical methods and practicum in speech-language pathology* (6th ed.). Plural Publishing.

Hegde, M. N., & Pomaville, F. (2022). *Assessment of communication disorders in children* (4th ed.). Plural Publishing.

Selected Books on Writing

Many excellent sources on general, technical, and professional writing are available. Students may consult the following books:

American Psychological Association. (2020). *Publication manual of the American Psychological Association* (7th ed.).

Bates, J. D. (2000). *Writing with precision.* Penguin Books.

Burchfield, R. W. (1996). *The new Fowler's modern English usage* (3rd ed.). Oxford University Press.

Butterfield, J. (2015). *Fowler's dictionary of modern English usage* (4th ed.). Oxford University Press.

Christiansen, S., Iverson, C., Flanagin, A., Livingston, E. H., Fischer, L., Manno, C., Gregoline, B., Frey, T., Fontanarosa, P. B., & Young, R. K. (2020). *AMA manual of style: A guide for authors and editors* (11th ed.). Oxford University Press.

Follett, W. (1998). *Modern American usage: A guide* (1st Rev. ed.). Hill & Wang.

Kane, T. S. (1988). *The new Oxford guide to writing.* Oxford University Press.

Kirszner, L. G., & Mandell, S. R. (2002). *The Holt handbook* (6th ed.). Harcourt College.

Modern Language Association. (2021). *MLA handbook* (9th ed.).

Morris, W., & Morris, M. (1992). *Harper dictionary of contemporary usage* (2nd ed.). Harper and Row.

Newman, E. (1976). *A civil tongue.* Bobbs-Merrill.

Strunk, W., Jr., & White, E. B. (1999). *The elements of style* (4th ed.). Pearson.

Thomas, F., & Turner, M. (1994). *Clear and simple as the truth: Writing classic prose*. Princeton University Press.

University of Chicago. (2017). *The Chicago manual of style* (17th ed.). University of Chicago Press.

Zinsser, W. (1980). *On writing well: An informal guide to writing nonfiction* (2nd ed.). Harper & Row.

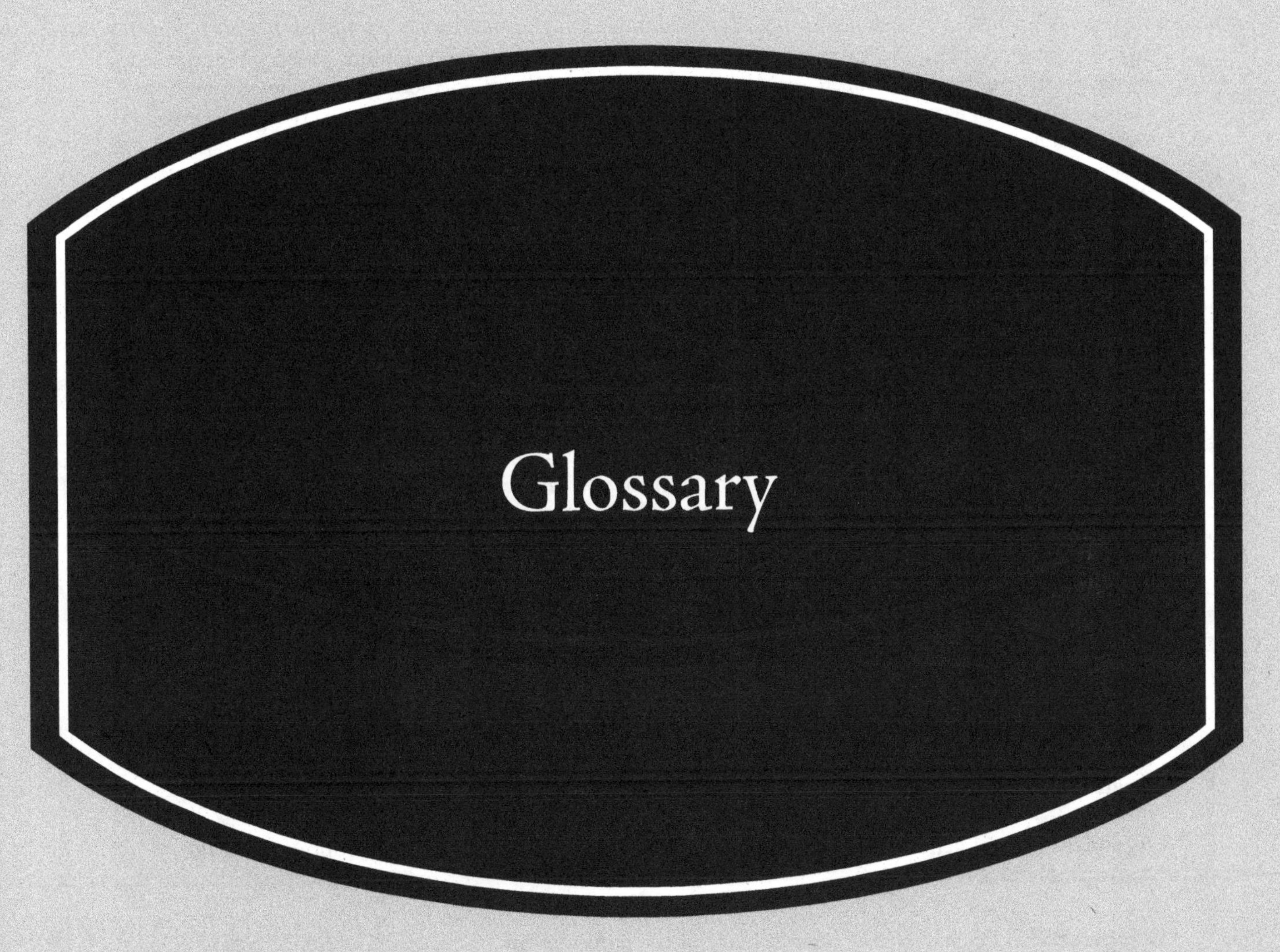

Glossary

In composing your scientific and professional writing, use the terms as defined in this glossary or as defined by your instructor or clinical supervisor. Also, consult books on clinical methods that your instructors and clinical supervisors recommend. Please note that many terms have other meanings in everyday discourse and writing; only the meanings relevant to the types of writing described in this book are given.

Ableism: Prejudice against people with physical disabilities; belief that able-bodied people are superior to people with disability.

Abstract: A brief summary of a research paper manuscript printed on a separate page (page 2); in the published report, the abstract is printed on the title page, below the authors' names and their affiliation.

Adultism: Discrimination against children and adolescents; a form of ageism.

African: Person living in Africa; not a synonym for *African American*; specificity is preferred (e.g., *Nigerian, Ethiopian* or *Nigerian American, Ethiopian American*).

African American: People of African background or ancestry who live in the United States; *Black* is an accepted alternative; *Afro-American* is outdated; *Negro* is offensive.

Aged: An outdated term for older persons.

Ageism: Stereotyping and discriminating against persons who are old; similar to *racism*.

Ageist: Similar to *racist*; the practice of, or the one who practices, ageism.

Agender: Lack of gender or gender neutral; may or may not be asexual; for pronouns, ask the person.

Ampersand: The character & used in place of the conjunction *and*; used in reference lists to connect names; not used in regular text except for inside parentheses for multiple authors.

Appendixes: Materials placed at the end of a paper or a chapter to give additional details on selected aspects of what is written in the body of the paper; the preferred plural spelling is appendixes, not appendices.

Arabic numerals: The widely used numbering system (e.g., 0, 1 through 9) in many parts of the world including most countries in Europe and the United States; also known as Hindu-Arabic numerals because of their origin in India; contrasted with roman numerals; the terms arabic and roman, when used to refer to number systems, are not capitalized except when they start a sentence.

Asexual: A person who experiences little or no sexual and romantic attraction toward any person.

Asian American: Person of Asian background or ancestry living in the United States; not a synonym for the *Asian* who lives in Asia; specificity is preferred (e.g., *Chinese American, Sri Lankan American, Korean American, Indian American*, etc.).

Assessment: Clinical procedures designed to diagnose a disorder or evaluate a client's existing and deficient communication behaviors and problems, and potential factors associated with them.

Audism: Prejudice against people with hearing loss; belief that people with typical hearing are superior to those with hearing loss.

Baselines: Measures of communication or other behaviors before the treatment is started; they help evaluate the client's improvement in treatment; they may be taken on evoked and modeled trials or in conversational speech. Baselines and baserates can both be nouns, but only baserate can be used as a verb (baserated, not baselined). Baselines of speech-language behaviors may be established by either using discrete trials or by taking conversational speech and language samples. See **Discrete baseline trial**.

Bibliography: A comprehensive list of publications on a given topic; not the same as a reference list; not attached to a paper or a chapter; may be free-standing; the format may be the same as that of a reference list.

Binary: Either male or female in the gender-related literature.

Bisexual: A person whose sexual and romantic attraction may extend to persons of the same gender or those of other genders.

Black or White people: The only two groups of people who may be identified by their skin color; people of any other color not to be identified in this manner (e.g., do not write *brown people*).

Block quotation: A quotation of 40 or more words reproduced verbatim from another source, including the author's own words published elsewhere; does not contain quotation marks and is set as a separate paragraph with a rigidly specified format.

Booster treatment: Treatment given any time after the client is dismissed from the original treatment to maintain clinically established skills; given after a follow-up assessment indicates a need for additional treatment.

Caucasian: An outdated term for the *White* or the *White European*; not to be used.

Chicana/Chicano: Persons of Mexican origin or ancestry; gendered; may be called Hispanics, but not all Hispanics are Chicana/o.

Cisgender: A person whose gender identity and sexual orientation are consistent with the sex assigned at birth; most people are *cisfemale* or *cismale*.

Clichés: Popular, overused, and dull expressions.

Conditioned generalized reinforcers: Tokens, money, and such other reinforcers that are effective in a wide range of conditions and are not subjected to satiation effect; in therapy, tokens may be exchanged for a variety of back-up reinforcers.

Conditioned reinforcers: Events that reinforce behaviors because of past learning experiences; same as secondary reinforcers.

Continuous reinforcement: A schedule in which the clinician reinforces all correct responses.

Conversational turn taking: Switching from the role of a speaker to that of a listener and vice versa; a conversational skill taught to persons with language disorders.

Copyediting: Editing of a manuscript by the publisher's editor for clarity, style, coverage, and so forth; the editor also may process the manuscript for typesetting.

Corrective feedback: Consequences that decrease behaviors; for example, saying "No," "Not correct," "Wrong," and so forth when a client's response is unacceptable.

Criteria: Rules to make various clinical judgments including when to model, when to stop modeling, and when a behavior is trained (e.g., the target is 90% correct production of the regular plural *s* in words).

Cross-dresser: A person who partially or fully dresses like a person belonging to a gender other than what was assigned at birth; does not imply a particular sexual orientation; replaces *transvestite*.

Deaf: A preferred, capitalized term by those who belong to the Deaf Culture and use a variety of sign languages.

Demisexual: A person who is not sexually attracted to someone unless also emotionally attracted or bonded.

Diagnostic report: A report on the methods and results of an assessment done on a client with a potential disorder or disease; description of diagnostic procedures and their results; also known as an *assessment report*.

Discrete baseline trial: An opportunity to produce a target response when no reinforcers or corrective feedback is given; may be modeled or evoked; steps are the same as those described under discrete training trial, evoked and discrete training trial, modeled except that no reinforcement or corrective feedback is provided for the correct and incorrect responses, respectively; the client may be periodically reinforced for being cooperative and responsive; used to determine the target response rate before introducing treatment.

Discrete training trial, evoked: An opportunity to produce a target response when the clinician does not model that response; in administering an evoked trial, you may:

- Place the stimulus item in front of the client or demonstrate the action or event with the help of objects.
- Ask the predetermined question (e.g., "What is this?").
- Wait a few seconds for the client to respond.
- Reinforce the correct response immediately (verbal praise or a tangible reinforcer).
- Give corrective feedback for incorrect responses.
- Record the response on the recording sheet.
- Pull the stimulus item toward yourself or remove it from the client's view.

- Wait a few seconds to mark the end of the trial.
- Initiate the next trial.

Discrete training trial, modeled: An opportunity to produce a target response when the clinician models that response; in administering a modeled trial, you may:

- Place the stimulus item in front of the client or demonstrate the action or event with the help of objects.
- Ask the predetermined question.
- Model the correct response immediately.
- Wait a few seconds for the client to respond.
- Reinforce the correct response immediately (verbal praise or a tangible reinforcer).
- Give corrective feedback for incorrect responses immediately.
- Record the response on the recording sheet.
- Pull the stimulus item toward yourself or remove it from the client's view.
- Wait a few seconds to mark the end of the trial.
- Initiate the next trial.

Elderly: An outdated term for the older person.

Electronic editing: Revising manuscript in such a way as to show the original and subsequent versions of the document on a computer screen; interactive method of manuscript processing by two or more individuals who review, comment, and respond to each other's revisions and comments.

Electronic manuscript submission: Preparation and submission of manuscripts as computer files, not as printed papers; journal articles and conference presentations typically submitted on a dedicated website maintained by the journal or an organization.

Electronic proofreading: Reading and correcting typeset digital manuscripts; typically, in the PDF format.

Email (e-mail): Electronic mail; sending messages electronically, via a network of computers.

Ethnicity: Shared language, culture, beliefs, and behavior patterns that help identify a group of people; not a synonym of *race*.

Euphemism: Hiding negative meanings by positive-sounding words; for example, the term *residentially challenged* is a positive-sounding term for the homeless.

Evoked trial: A structured opportunity to produce a response when the clinician does not model; presenting a picture and asking a question (e.g., "What is this?") is an example of an evoking trial.

Exemplar: A response that illustrates a target behavior (e.g., *These are two cups* is an exemplar of the regular plural *s*).

Fading: A method of reducing the controlling power of a stimulus while still maintaining the response.

Fixed interval schedule: An intermittent schedule of reinforcement in which a response produced after a fixed duration is reinforced.

Fixed ratio schedule: An intermittent schedule of reinforcement in which a certain number of responses are required to earn a reinforcer.

Flush left: Typing the first character flush with the left margin, with no indentation.

Follow-up: Probe or assessment of response maintenance after dismissal from treatment; usually involves taking a new speech and language sample to assess the production of previously taught responses or skills.

Footers: A feature of computer word processors; a full or abbreviated title of a paper or a chapter automatically printed at the bottom of a page; may contain other information such as the chapter number, time and date of printing, and the author name; may be flush-left, centered, or right-aligned; not used in the style of the *Publication Manual of the American Psychological Association.*

FTP: File Transfer Protocol; electronic means of transferring data from one computer to another via a network of computers.

Functional outcome: Generalized, broader, and socially and personally meaningful effects of treatment; an overall improvement in communication between clients, their families, and their caregivers.

Gay men: Persons who are sexually and romantically attracted to individuals of the same sex and gender.

Gender: Feelings and behaviors a society or culture associates with the biological sex of a person; a social identity construct.

Gender-affirming surgery: Surgical modification of a person's body to make it consistent with that person's gender identity; also called *gender-confirming* or *sex reassignment* surgery; not all transgender people will have undergone this surgery; replaces *sex change operation*, a term not to be used.

Gender binary: The concept that gender can only be female or male and should behave as society expects; prejudicial term.

Gender diversity: Varied gender identities; an umbrella term that includes different gender identities; some may prefer this to *gender nonbinary* or *gender nonconforming.*

Gender dysphoria: Distress caused by an incongruence between a person's felt or expressed gender and the social role expected on the basis of sex assigned at birth. A controversial psychiatric diagnostic term from the *Diagnostic and Statistical Manual of Mental Disorders* (5th ed.; *DSM-5*); replaces *gender identity disorder.*

Gender expression: Gender-related overt behaviors including appearance (e.g., clothing and hairstyle), speech, voice, personal pronoun usage, and general behavior. Gender expression and gender identity may or may not be identical.

Gender-fluid: Variable gender identity across time.

Gender identity: Self-description of one's gender and pronoun and a pattern of behavior consistent with that description; deeply felt feelings about one's sense of being a person of certain gender, no fixed gender, or no gender (agender); may be binary (girl, boy, man, woman) or nonbinary (genderqueer, gender-fluid, gender-nonconforming, transgender, two-spirit, etc.); may be consistent with sex assigned at birth or at variance.

Gender nonconfirming: Persons whose gender-related behaviors are inconsistent with social expectations; not a synonym for *transgender*.

Genderqueer: Persons whose gender expressions are somewhere in between the male–female identity, totally outside of male–female identities, or with their own unique identities; not a synonym for *transgender*, although may be used as an umbrella term for varied gender identities.

Generalized production of target responses: Production of responses when the treatment procedure is not in effect; for example, the clinician may take a speech sample without implementing any treatment procedures to see if a child who has been taught various language structures uses them; this procedure of assessing generalized production is called a probe.

Headers: An abbreviated or full title of a paper, chapter, and the page number automatically printed on top of each page of a manuscript; may be flush left, centered, or right-aligned; in the APA style, typed right-aligned; contrasts with footers.

Headings: Subtitles within a paper or a chapter that suggest the subtopic that follows; classified into levels (e.g., Level 1 and Level 2 headings); not to be confused with a title, headers, page headers (of a manuscript), or running heads.

Hearing loss: Hearing acuity reduced to varying degrees; preferable to *hearing impairment*.

Heterosexism: A belief that heterosexual behavior is normal; refers to prejudice and discriminatory behavior toward those with diverse sexual orientation.

Hispanic: Geographically dispersed and culturally varied people of Spanish language background; not a race; preferable to be specific (e.g., *Mexican American*, *Cuban American*, *Chilean American*).

Homoprejudice: Prejudicial beliefs and behaviors toward lesbians and gay men; also called *homonegativity* and *homophobia*.

Homosexuality: Sexual attraction felt toward persons of the same sex and gender; an outdated and prejudicial term because of the past legal sanctions and implications of pathology.

Identity-first language: Describing disability by starting with the disability itself; person comes next (e.g., *Deaf person*, not *the person who is deaf*; *autistic person*, not *the person with autism*); to be used only when the persons in question prefer it as a matter of personal and sociocultural pride; see *Person-first language*.

IEPs: Individual educational programs for children with disabilities or special needs; typically written in educational settings; similar to target behaviors and treatment procedures specified in clinical settings.

IFSPs: Individualized family service plans developed for infants and toddlers and their family members; typically written in educational settings.

Imitation: Learning in which responses take the same form as their stimuli; modeling provides the stimuli; often necessary in the initial stages of treatment.

Informant: A person who gives case history and related information to the clinician; it may be the client themself or another person (e.g., a family member).

Initial response: The first, simplified component of a target response used in shaping a more complex reponse.

Instructions: Verbal stimuli that gain control over other persons' actions; description of how to perform certain actions; often given before modeling a skill for the client.

Intellectual disability: Persons with deficits in reasoning, abstract thinking, and academic learning; with deficits in such adaptive functions as personal independence and social responsibility; observed during the developmental period; replaces the term *mental retardation*.

Intermediate response: Responses other than the initial and final, used in shaping.

Intermittent reinforcement: Reinforcing only some responses or responses produced with some delay between reinforcers.

Intermixed probes: Procedures of assessing generalized production by alternating trained and untrained stimulus items on discrete trials; one trial involves a previously trained stimulus (e.g., the picture of two cups, used in training the plural *s*), and the next trial involves an untrained (novel) stimulus (e.g., the picture of two books, not used in training); correct responses given to untrained stimuli are counted to calculate the percentage correct probe response rate. See also **Probe** and **Pure probes**.

Internet: A high-speed digital network to transfer data through standard communication protocols between computers linked locally, nationally, and globally.

Intersex: Anatomic and biological (e.g., chromosomal patterns) sex characteristics that do not permit a binary classification of male or female; ambiguity may be present at birth or may emerge later, often at puberty.

Latin@: People of Latin American ancestry; varied pronunciation including /lətinaʊ/; another gender-neutral term like *Latinx.*

Latino/Latina: Gendered terms for the people of Latin American (including Brazilian) origin or ancestry; also spelled Latina/o or Latino/a; not a synonym for *Hispanic*; specificity is preferred (e.g., Chilean, Cuban, Bolivian, Mexican); ascertain the personal preference.

Latinx: People of Latin American background or descent; gender-neutral because it replaces the gendered *o* or *a*; hence accepted by the LGBTQIA+ communities.

Lesbian: A woman who is sexually and romantically attracted to persons of the same sex and gender.

LGBTQIA+: Lesbian, Gay, Bisexual, Transgender, Queer/Questioning, Intersex, Asexual, and More; an umbrella term, still evolving, for people whose self-identified gender identity, sexual orientation, or both are outside of the cisgender heteronormative constructs.

Maintenance strategy: Extension of treatment to natural settings; a collection of methods to help maintain clinically established skills over time; includes such procedures as teaching the client to self-monitor their behaviors and training significant others to prompt and reinforce those behaviors in natural settings.

Manual guidance: Physical guidance provided to shape a response; taking the client's hand and pointing to a correct picture is an example.

Mean length of utterance (MLU): A measure of language development; measured as the number of morphemes or words in each utterance and averaged across a collection of utterances.

Misogyny: Hatred of women and girls; may lead to violence against them; an extreme form of sexism.

Modeled trial: An opportunity to imitate a response when the clinician models it; see **Discrete trial, modeled.**

Modeling: The clinician's production of the target response the client is expected to learn; used to teach imitation (e.g., showing the picture of an apple, and asking, "What is this?" and immediately modeling the response "Say, apple.").

Mood: In grammar, mood refers to various verb forms that indicate whether implied or expressed actions are more or less likely; indicative mood expresses factual statements; subjunctive mood suggests uncertainty; and imperative mood suggests a command or request.

Native American: Indigenous people of the Americas; often used as the native people of the United States or Canada; may be preferable to *American Indian* to avoid confusion with people of India or Indian heritage (*Indian Americans*); specificity is preferred (e.g., *Navajo, Cherokee, Shoshone*); *people* or *nation* but not *tribe.*

Negative reinforcers: Aversive events that are removed, reduced, postponed, or prevented by specific responses; such responses then increase in frequency. See also **Positive reinforcers.**

Nonbinary: Refers to a range of gender identities that does not conform to the categorical male–female identity; some may prefer *gender diversity*.

Online: A format of storing information that can be retrieved in an interactive manner; many journals now are online, meaning that they can be searched through the internet.

Operational definitions: Scientific definitions that describe how what is defined is measured; clinical treatment targets should be defined operationally (e.g., "I will teach language competence" is not an operational description of a target; "I will teach the following four grammatical morphemes in sentences" followed by a list, is).

Oriental: An outdated term for the people of the Eastern hemisphere; pejorative because it has discriminatory colonial connotations and mainly includes objects considered exotic (e.g., carpets, furniture, decorative art).

Orofacial examination: A visual examination of the oral and facial structures to detect gross abnormality; includes several tasks (such as producing certain vowels, moving the tongue, lifting the soft palate) to assess functional integrity of the oral and facial structures; also known as oral-peripheral examination.

Page header: A briefer title of the article, printed on the upper-right corner of each page of the article except for those containing figures; not to be confused with the running head.

Pansexual: Persons who feel sexually attracted to people of all genders and sexes.

Parallelism: Expressing similar ideas or a series of ideas in similar forms; expressing similar ideas or a series of ideas in different forms violates parallelism, resulting in nonparallel constructions.

Parenthetic constructions: Phrases within sentences that express ideas that are not integral to those sentences; enclosed within parentheses.

PDF: Portable Document Format; a method of converting documents prepared on various computer platforms and operating systems into a single format, often before printing them; when PDFs are exchanged across computers, the original and the converted formats are retained.

Peer training: Training peers of clients to evoke and reinforce target behaviors in natural settings; a maintenance strategy.

People of color: Acceptable alternative to *non-White people*; *underrepresented groups* is also acceptable, but *minorities* is not because it is nonspecific; *minorities* may be inaccurate as well because in some regions, non-Whites may be a majority.

Person-first language: Describing disability by starting with the person (e.g., *person with traumatic brain injury, child with language disorder*); see **Identity-first language**.

Positive reinforcers: Events that, when presented immediately after a response is made, increase the future probability of that response. See also **Negative reinforcers**.

Pragmatic features: Aspects of language use in social contexts; targets of language treatment; pragmatic language targets for treatment include skills such as conversational turn taking and topic maintenance.

Primary reinforcers: Unconditioned reinforcers whose effects do not depend on past learning (e.g., food).

Probe: Procedure to assess generalized production of responses. See also **Intermixed probes** and **Pure probes**.

Probe criterion: A rule that says that a trained response is satisfactorily produced without the treatment variables; for example, 95% fluency maintained in conversational speech when the clinician does not reinforce or prompt the target fluency describes a probe criterion.

Prompts: Special stimuli that increase the probability of a response; prompts may be verbal or nonverbal; similar to hints.

Proofs: Also known as page proofs; the typeset manuscript sent to the author for final review; previously printed, and currently, in the PDF format.

Pure probes: Procedures for assessing generalized production with only untrained stimulus items; contrasted with intermixed probes in which trained and untrained stimuli are alternated; for example, in administering pure probes, a clinician may present 20 untrained pictures that show plural objects to assess whether the child will produce the plural *s* without reinforcement.

Queer: Originally used to belittle and demean the community of lesbian, gay, bisexual, and transsexual individuals, now many in the same community have reclaimed the word for their own designation as a matter of pride; not all members of this community may accept the term, so it is essential to ask the person for preference.

Questioning: Individuals who are exploring their gender identity and sexual orientation because of uncertainty.

Race: People who share a set of physical features and consider those features socially and culturally significant; terms that refer to racial differences include the *Aboriginal, African American, White, Asian, Native American, Pacific Islander, Native Hawaiian*, and so forth; capitalized because they are proper nouns; see **Ethnicity**.

Reference list: A list of all and only the works cited in the body of text; follows a prescribed format; always attached to a paper, a chapter, or an entire book; not free-standing; not to be confused with a bibliography.

Reinforcers: Events that follow behaviors and thereby increase the future probability of those behaviors. See also **Positive** and **Negative reinforcers**.

Response cost: A method of directly reducing an undesirable behavior by presenting a reinforcer for a desirable (alternative) behavior (e.g., fluent speech) and withdrawing a reinforcer for every undesirable behavior (e.g., stuttered speech).

Right-justification: Printing lines to align with the right margin, as in most printed books; when computer printed, the words may have uneven spaces between them; not accepted in the APA style.

Running head: An abbreviated title of a research paper printed flush-left at the top of the title page, but below the page header; printed in all capitals; it does not exceed 50 character spaces including letters, punctuation marks, and spaces between letters.

Schedules of reinforcement: Different patterns of reinforcement that generate different patterns of responses; includes such schedules as continuous reinforcement (every response is reinforced) and intermittent reinforcement (some responses are not reinforced).

Self-control: A behavior that monitors other behaviors of the same person; a maintenance strategy; clients who are taught to count their errors, for example, have learned to monitor their responses.

Senile: An outdated term for persons with *dementia*.

Serial comma: The comma that is used in a series of similar elements including before *and* and *or*, as in *clients, their families, and employers*; *roses, gardenias, or magnolias*.

Sex: Assigned male or female category at the time of birth, based on external anatomy; more biological than the personally and socially constructed *gender identity*, which may or may not align with assigned sex.

Sex assignment at birth: What the birth certificate says about the sex of the individual.

Sexism: Discriminatory behavior toward women and girls; may lead to violence against women and girls; in clinical and scientific writing, inappropriate use of male pronouns and other writing styles perpetuate sexism.

Sexual orientation: A set of blended emotional, romantic, sexual, affectional, and social behaviors that imply sexual attraction or nonattraction to other persons; part of a person's gender and personal identity; replaces *sexual preference*.

Shaping: A method of teaching nonexistent responses that are not even imitated. The responses are simplified and taught in an ascending sequence. Also known as successive approximations.

Significant others: People who are important in the lives of clients; includes family members, peers, colleagues, and teachers; training them in prompting and reinforcing a client's target behavior is a maintenance strategy.

SOAP notes: Subjective, objective, assessment, and plan; brief progress reports more commonly written in medical settings.

Social reinforcers: A variety of conditioned reinforcers, which include verbal praise.

Straight: Persons who are sexually attracted to members of another sex.

Subscript: A character or a number printed lower than the rest of the printed line; the 1 in X_1 is a subscript character.

Superscript: A character or a number printed higher than the rest of the printed line; the d in S^d is a superscript character.

Targets: Behaviors a client is taught; communication skills that are trained.

Terminal response: The final response targeted in shaping.

Time-out: A period of nonreinforcement imposed response, contingently; the typical effect is reduced rate of that response.

Title: The name given to a paper or a chapter; printed on the title page; repeated on every page of a book chapter; printed, in an abbreviated form, on all pages of a research paper; not to be confused with headings in a paper or chapter.

Tokens: Objects that are earned during treatment and exchanged later for back-up reinforcers.

Topic maintenance: Talking on a single topic for an extended period of time; a language skill taught to persons with language disorders.

Training criterion: A rule that says that a given target response has been trained; for example, 90% correct responses over a block of trials for a given target response may mean that the response has been trained.

Transgender: A person whose gender identity and gender-related behaviors differ from the conventional expectations based on their sex assignment at birth; may or may not have undergone gender-affirming surgery; adjective, not a noun.

Transition: A personal (speech, dress), medical (hormonal, surgical), and legal (name change) process of altering one's sex assigned at birth; replaces *sex change*.

Transprejudice: Discriminatory behavior toward transgender; the same as *transnegativity*.

Transsexual: Persons who have transitioned through medical intervention; an older term; most people prefer to call themselves *transgender*.

Treatment: Management of contingent relations between antecedents, responses, and consequences; rearrangement of verbal interactions between a speaker and their listener.

Trial: A structured opportunity to produce a response; see **Discrete training trial, evoked** and **Discrete training trial, modeled**.

Two-spirit: Persons with more than one sexual identity, such as both a male and a female identity; may feel a same-sex or any other-sex attraction; a Native American term.

Underprivileged: People with less money, education, resources, and political power; may be of any race, color, national origin, or ancestry; not a generic term for racial groups or minorities.

Variable interval schedule: An intermittent reinforcement schedule in which the time duration between reinforcers is varied around an average.

Variable ratio schedule: An intermittent reinforcement schedule in which the number of responses needed to earn a reinforcer is varied around an average.

Vocal wetness: An impression that the voice is wet, often noticed in patients with dysphagia and is due to pharyngeal residue of food or liquid.

World Wide Web (WWW): A vast digital structure of interconnected computers that stores electronic files of data that can be retrieved and transmitted across the internet; a digital-graphical environment for creating, storing, and sharing information.

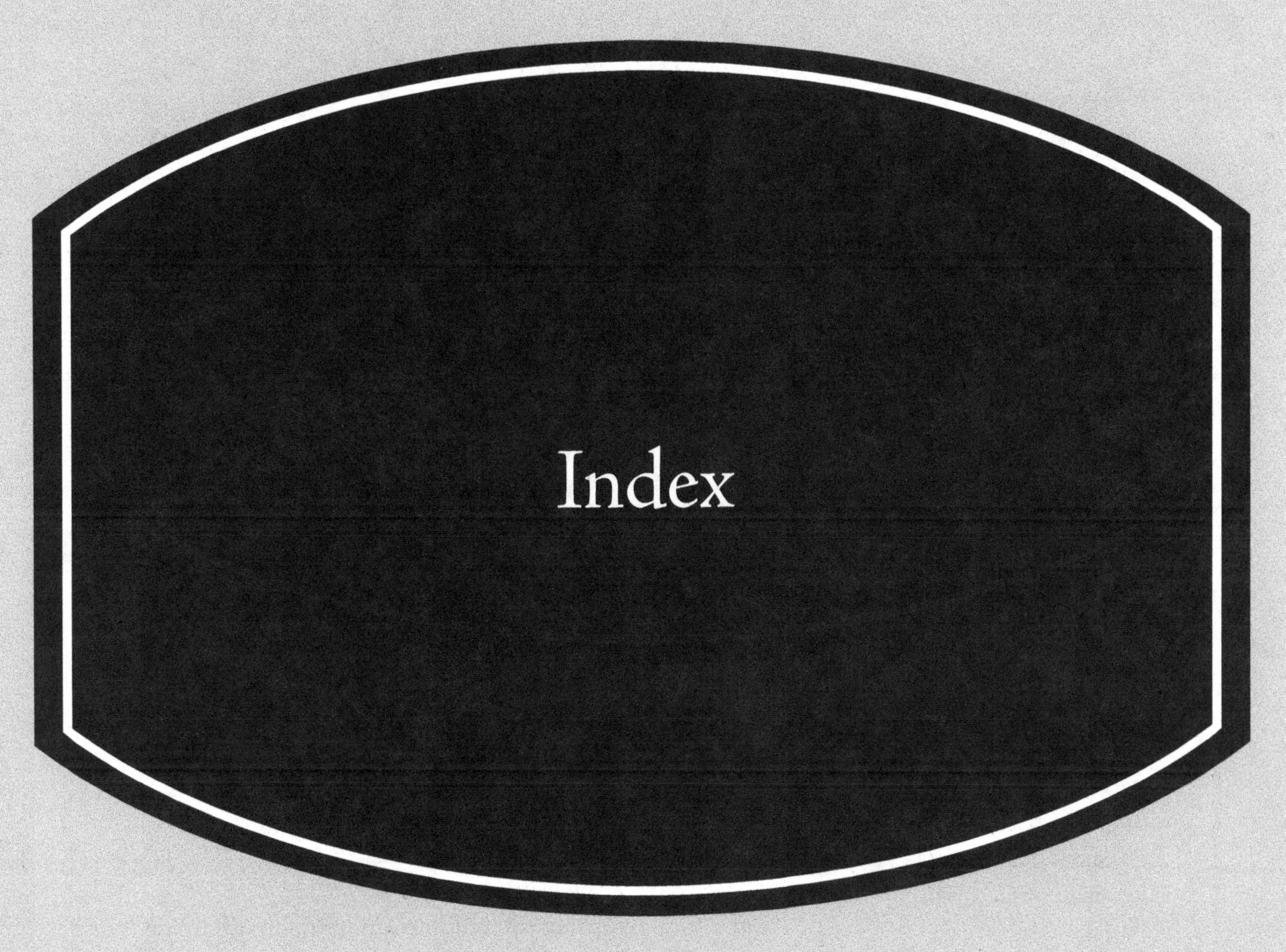
Index

A

B

C

D

N

O

P

Q

R

S